Practice the RMA!

Registered Medical Assistant Practice Questions

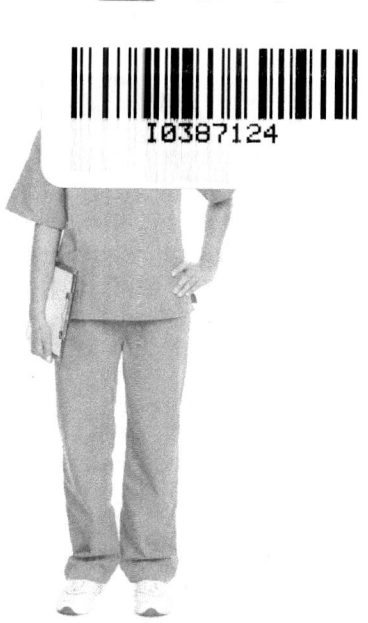

Published by

Complete TEST Preparation Inc.

Copyright © 2011 Complete Test Preparation Inc. ALL RIGHTS RESERVED.

No part of this book may be reproduced or transferred in any form or by any means, graphic, electronic, or mechanical, including photocopying, recording, web distribution, taping, or by any information storage retrieval system, without the written permission of the author.

Notice: Complete Test Preparation Inc. makes every reasonable effort to obtain from reliable sources accurate, complete, and timely information about the subjects covered in this book. Nevertheless, changes can be made in the tests or the administration of the tests at any time and Complete Test Preparation Inc. makes no representation or warranty of any kind, either expressed or implied as to the accuracy, timeliness, reliability, suitability or availability with respect to the information contained in this document for any purpose. Any reliance you place on such information is therefore strictly at your own risk.

Disclaimer

The author(s) shall not be liable for any loss incurred as a consequence of the use and application, directly or indirectly, of any information presented in this work. Sold with the understanding, the author is not engaged in rendering professional services or advice. If advice or expert assistance is required, the services of a competent professional should be sought.

Complete Test Preparation Inc. and the author(s) shall have neither liability nor responsibility to any person or entity with respect to any loss or damages arising form the information contained in this book.

The company, product and service names used in this publication are for identification purposes only. All trademarks and registered trademarks are the property of their respective owners. Complete Test Preparation Inc. is not affiliated with any educational institution. Use of a term in this book should not be regarded as affecting the validity of any trademark or service mark.

We strongly recommend that students check with exam providers for up-to-date information regarding test content.

The RMA and Registered Medical Assistant are registered trademarks of the National Association for Health Professionals, Inc., who are not involved in the production of, and do not endorse this book.

ISBN-13: 978-1-77245-051-4

Version 6.5 June 2015

Published by
Complete Test Preparation Inc.
Victoria BC Canada
Visit us on the web at http://www.test-preparation.ca
Printed in the USA

About Complete Test Preparation Inc.

Complete Test Preparation Inc. has been publishing high quality study materials since 2005. Thousands of students visit our websites every year, and thousands of students, teachers and parents all over the world have purchased our teaching materials, curriculum, study guides and practice tests.

Complete Test Preparation Inc. is committed to providing students with the best study materials and practice tests available on the market. Members of our team combine years of teaching experience, with experienced writers and editors, all with advanced degrees (Masters or higher).

Feedback

We Welcome your comments! You can email us (feedback@test-preparation.ca) and let us know what you think! We will carefully review your comments and may include them in future revisions.

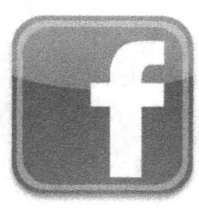 **Find us on Facebook**

www.facebook.com/CompleteTestPreparation

Contents

Getting Started	**6**
What is on the RMA	6
Practice Test 1	**7**
Answer Key	71
Practice Test 2	**107**
Answer Key	169
Pharmacy Dosage Problems	**197**
Answer Key	202

Getting Started

CONGRATULATIONS! By deciding to take the Registered Medical Assistant Exam (RMA), you have taken the first step toward a great future! Of course, there is no point in taking this important examination unless you intend to do your very best in order to earn the highest grade you possibly can. That means getting yourself organized and discovering the best approaches, methods and strategies to master the material. Yes, that will require real effort and dedication on your part but if you are willing to focus your energy and devote the study time necessary, before you know it you will be opening that letter of acceptance for the job of your dreams.

We know that taking on a new endeavour can be a little scary, and it is easy to feel unsure of where to begin. That's where we come in. This study guide is designed to help you improve your test-taking skills, show you a few tricks of the trade and increase both your competency and confidence.

What is on the RMA

The RMA has three sections: General Medical Assisting Knowledge, Administrative Medical Assisting, and Clinical Medical Assisting.

General Medical Assisting Knowledge 41%

This section covers anatomy and physiology, medical terminology, medical law, medical ethics, human relations (communication), and patient education

Administrative Medical Assisting 24%

This section covers insurance, coding and claims, and finance and bookkeeping.

Clinical Medical Assisting 35%

This section covers, asepsis, sterilization, vital signs, clinical pharmacology, minor surgery, therapeutic modalities, laboratory procedures, and electrocardiography (ECG).

Practice Test Questions Set 1

The questions below are not the same as you will find on the RMA - that would be too easy! And nobody knows what the questions will be and they change all the time. Below are general questions that cover the same subject areas as the RMA. So, while the format and exact wording of the questions may differ slightly, and change from year to year, if you can answer the questions below, you will have no problem with the RMA.

For the best results, take these Practice Test Questions as if it were the real exam. Set aside time when you will not be disturbed, and a location that is quiet and free of distractions. Read the instructions carefully, read each question carefully, and answer to the best of your ability.

Use the bubble answer sheets provided. When you have completed the Practice Questions, check your answer against the Answer Key and read the explanation provided.

Do not attempt more than one set of practice test questions in one day. After completing the first practice test, wait two or three days before attempting the second set of questions.

Part I – General Medical Assisting Knowledge

Section I – Anatomy and Physiology

1. A B C D
2. A B C D
3. A B C D
4. A B C D
5. A B C D
6. A B C D
7. A B C D
8. A B C D
9. A B C D
10. A B C D
11. A B C D
12. A B C D
13. A B C D
14. A B C D
15. A B C D
16. A B C D
17. A B C D
18. A B C D
19. A B C D
20. A B C D
21. A B C D
22. A B C D
23. A B C D
24. A B C D
25. A B C D
26. A B C D
27. A B C D
28. A B C D
29. A B C D
30. A B C D
31. A B C D
32. A B C D
33. A B C D
34. A B C D
35. A B C D
36. A B C D
37. A B C D
38. A B C D
39. A B C D
40. A B C D
41. A B C D
42. A B C D
43. A B C D
44. A B C D
45. A B C D
46. A B C D
47. A B C D
48. A B C D
49. A B C D
50. A B C D

Section II – Medical Terminology

1. A B C D
2. A B C D
3. A B C D
4. A B C D
5. A B C D
6. A B C D
7. A B C D
8. A B C D
9. A B C D
10. A B C D

11. A B C D
12. A B C D
13. A B C D
14. A B C D
15. A B C D
16. A B C D
17. A B C D
18. A B C D
19. A B C D
20. A B C D

21. A B C D
22. A B C D
23. A B C D
24. A B C D

Section III – Medical Law and Ethics

1. Ⓐ Ⓑ Ⓒ Ⓓ   11. Ⓐ Ⓑ Ⓒ Ⓓ   21. Ⓐ Ⓑ Ⓒ Ⓓ
2. Ⓐ Ⓑ Ⓒ Ⓓ   12. Ⓐ Ⓑ Ⓒ Ⓓ   22. Ⓐ Ⓑ Ⓒ Ⓓ
3. Ⓐ Ⓑ Ⓒ Ⓓ   13. Ⓐ Ⓑ Ⓒ Ⓓ   23. Ⓐ Ⓑ Ⓒ Ⓓ
4. Ⓐ Ⓑ Ⓒ Ⓓ   14. Ⓐ Ⓑ Ⓒ Ⓓ   24. Ⓐ Ⓑ Ⓒ Ⓓ
5. Ⓐ Ⓑ Ⓒ Ⓓ   15. Ⓐ Ⓑ Ⓒ Ⓓ   25. Ⓐ Ⓑ Ⓒ Ⓓ
6. Ⓐ Ⓑ Ⓒ Ⓓ   16. Ⓐ Ⓑ Ⓒ Ⓓ
7. Ⓐ Ⓑ Ⓒ Ⓓ   17. Ⓐ Ⓑ Ⓒ Ⓓ
8. Ⓐ Ⓑ Ⓒ Ⓓ   18. Ⓐ Ⓑ Ⓒ Ⓓ
9. Ⓐ Ⓑ Ⓒ Ⓓ   19. Ⓐ Ⓑ Ⓒ Ⓓ
10. Ⓐ Ⓑ Ⓒ Ⓓ   20. Ⓐ Ⓑ Ⓒ Ⓓ

Section IV – Communication and Patient Education

1. Ⓐ Ⓑ Ⓒ Ⓓ   11. Ⓐ Ⓑ Ⓒ Ⓓ
2. Ⓐ Ⓑ Ⓒ Ⓓ   12. Ⓐ Ⓑ Ⓒ Ⓓ
3. Ⓐ Ⓑ Ⓒ Ⓓ   13. Ⓐ Ⓑ Ⓒ Ⓓ
4. Ⓐ Ⓑ Ⓒ Ⓓ   14. Ⓐ Ⓑ Ⓒ Ⓓ
5. Ⓐ Ⓑ Ⓒ Ⓓ   15. Ⓐ Ⓑ Ⓒ Ⓓ
6. Ⓐ Ⓑ Ⓒ Ⓓ   16. Ⓐ Ⓑ Ⓒ Ⓓ
7. Ⓐ Ⓑ Ⓒ Ⓓ   17. Ⓐ Ⓑ Ⓒ Ⓓ
8. Ⓐ Ⓑ Ⓒ Ⓓ   18. Ⓐ Ⓑ Ⓒ Ⓓ
9. Ⓐ Ⓑ Ⓒ Ⓓ   19. Ⓐ Ⓑ Ⓒ Ⓓ
10. Ⓐ Ⓑ Ⓒ Ⓓ   20. Ⓐ Ⓑ Ⓒ Ⓓ

Part II – Administrative Medical Assisting

1. A B C D
2. A B C D
3. A B C D
4. A B C D
5. A B C D
6. A B C D
7. A B C D
8. A B C D
9. A B C D
10. A B C D
11. A B C D
12. A B C D
13. A B C D
14. A B C D
15. A B C D
16. A B C D
17. A B C D
18. A B C D
19. A B C D
20. A B C D
21. A B C D
22. A B C D
23. A B C D
24. A B C D
25. A B C D
26. A B C D
27. A B C D
28. A B C D
29. A B C D
30. A B C D
31. A B C D
32. A B C D
33. A B C D
34. A B C D

Part III – Clinical Medical Assisting

1. Ⓐ Ⓑ Ⓒ Ⓓ
2. Ⓐ Ⓑ Ⓒ Ⓓ
3. Ⓐ Ⓑ Ⓒ Ⓓ
4. Ⓐ Ⓑ Ⓒ Ⓓ
5. Ⓐ Ⓑ Ⓒ Ⓓ
6. Ⓐ Ⓑ Ⓒ Ⓓ
7. Ⓐ Ⓑ Ⓒ Ⓓ
8. Ⓐ Ⓑ Ⓒ Ⓓ
9. Ⓐ Ⓑ Ⓒ Ⓓ
10. Ⓐ Ⓑ Ⓒ Ⓓ
11. Ⓐ Ⓑ Ⓒ Ⓓ
12. Ⓐ Ⓑ Ⓒ Ⓓ
13. Ⓐ Ⓑ Ⓒ Ⓓ
14. Ⓐ Ⓑ Ⓒ Ⓓ
15. Ⓐ Ⓑ Ⓒ Ⓓ
16. Ⓐ Ⓑ Ⓒ Ⓓ
17. Ⓐ Ⓑ Ⓒ Ⓓ
18. Ⓐ Ⓑ Ⓒ Ⓓ
19. Ⓐ Ⓑ Ⓒ Ⓓ
20. Ⓐ Ⓑ Ⓒ Ⓓ
21. Ⓐ Ⓑ Ⓒ Ⓓ
22. Ⓐ Ⓑ Ⓒ Ⓓ
23. Ⓐ Ⓑ Ⓒ Ⓓ
24. Ⓐ Ⓑ Ⓒ Ⓓ
25. Ⓐ Ⓑ Ⓒ Ⓓ
26. Ⓐ Ⓑ Ⓒ Ⓓ
27. Ⓐ Ⓑ Ⓒ Ⓓ
28. Ⓐ Ⓑ Ⓒ Ⓓ
29. Ⓐ Ⓑ Ⓒ Ⓓ
30. Ⓐ Ⓑ Ⓒ Ⓓ
31. Ⓐ Ⓑ Ⓒ Ⓓ
32. Ⓐ Ⓑ Ⓒ Ⓓ
33. Ⓐ Ⓑ Ⓒ Ⓓ
34. Ⓐ Ⓑ Ⓒ Ⓓ
35. Ⓐ Ⓑ Ⓒ Ⓓ
36. Ⓐ Ⓑ Ⓒ Ⓓ
37. Ⓐ Ⓑ Ⓒ Ⓓ
38. Ⓐ Ⓑ Ⓒ Ⓓ
39. Ⓐ Ⓑ Ⓒ Ⓓ
40. Ⓐ Ⓑ Ⓒ Ⓓ
41. Ⓐ Ⓑ Ⓒ Ⓓ
42. Ⓐ Ⓑ Ⓒ Ⓓ
43. Ⓐ Ⓑ Ⓒ Ⓓ
44. Ⓐ Ⓑ Ⓒ Ⓓ
45. Ⓐ Ⓑ Ⓒ Ⓓ

Part 1 – Anatomy & Physiology, Medical Terminology

1. Anatomy breaks the human abdomen down into segments called _____.

    a. Regions
    b. Districts
    c. Quadrants
    d. Areas

2. The quadrant that is largely responsible for digestion is _____.

    a. Left Upper
    b. Right Upper
    c. Right Left
    d. Left Lower

3. The body organ that is NOT located within the Right Upper Quadrant is _____.

    a. Liver
    b. Gall Bladder
    c. Duodenum
    d. Sigmoid colon

4. The organ that is located in the Right Lower Quadrant is _____.

    a. Appendix
    b. Heart
    c. Left lung
    d. Trachea

Practice Test Questions Set 1

5. One reason that medical professionals should know the names and locations of the Quadrant is _____.

   a. To keep the patient's condition a secret from him.

   b. To communicate about patients' conditions with other doctors and medical professionals.

   c. For insurance purposes.

   d. Not knowing the quadrants almost always results in death for the patient.

6. The stomach and colon are both in the _____.

   a. Left Upper Quadrant

   b. Right Upper Quadrant

   c. Right Lower Quadrant

   d. Left Lower Quadrant

7. Commonly used abbreviations for the Quadrants are _____.

   A. QUR, QUL, QLR, QLL

   B. ABC, DEF, GHI, JKL

   C. RUQ, LUQ, RLQ, LLQ

   D. RR, LL, CQ, RQ

8. The intestines are located in _____.

   a. LUQ

   b. LLQ

   c. RLQ

   d. All of the above

9. The stomach is located in _____.

    a. LLQ
    b. LUQ
    c. RUQ
    d. RLQ

10. The gallbladder is located in _____.

    a. RUQ
    b. LUQ
    c. LLQ
    d. RLQ

11. An example of human homeostasis is _____.

    a. Metabolism
    b. Adrenalin
    c. Hormones
    d. Fluid Balance

12. Human homeostasis is the ability of the body to regulate its _____ in response to fluctuations in the environment outside the body.

    a. Inner environment
    b. Outer environment
    c. Temperature
    d. Metabolism

13. The amount of energy / calories that your body requires to maintain itself is known as _____.

    a. Temperature
    b. Fluid balance
    c. Botulism
    d. Metabolism

14. An example of a person whose metabolism has lowered is _____.

    a. A woman who is in her teens and quite athletic
    b. A man who is past 30 and whose body is losing muscle.
    c. A man who is past 30 and works out daily.
    d. A man who is past 30 and eats a low-fat diet.

15. An example of something that increases a person's metabolism is _____.

    a. Aerobic exercise
    b. Mental exercise
    c. Eating a fatty diet
    d. Reading

16. Fluid balance might be negatively impacted when the _____ fail.

    a. Kidneys
    b. Ears
    c. Nose
    d. Legs

17. Fluid balance is important, because _____ comprises about 60-70% of a person's weight.

    a. Calcium
    b. Water
    c. Iron
    d. Bone

18. As a person moves from adolescence to adulthood, their metabolism _____.

    a. Begins to get higher
    b. Begins to get lower.
    c. Stabilizes
    d. Fluctuates wildly

19. "Met" refers to _____.

    a. Mitosis
    b. The person's heart rate
    c. The person's blood pressure
    d. The person's metabolic rate.

20. Fluid balance is important, because the human body loses water every day through urination, perspiration, feces, and _____.

    a. Breathing
    b. Resting
    c. Meditating
    d. Outbursts of temper

21. What is the smallest unit of life in our bodies?

    a. Atom
    b. Molecule
    c. Proton
    d. Cell

22. Name one function of the cell membrane.

    a. Divide into other cells.
    b. Control what moves into and out of the cell.
    c. Fight infection.
    d. Trap bacteria.

23. What is the process of a larger cell dividing into two or more smaller cells called?

    a. Cell division
    b. Cell multiplication
    c. Mitosis
    d. Metabolism

24. Prophase, metaphase, anaphase, and telophase are phases of _____.

    a. Cell division
    b. Infection
    c. Mitosis
    d. Adrenaline

25. Mitosis is a scientific term that, in layman's terms, means:

    a. Cellular disease.
    b. Nuclear cell division (division of the cell nucleus).
    c. Infection.
    d. Atomic fusion.

26. What is the stage of mitosis in which the chromatin condenses and becomes a chromosome?

    a. Prophase
    b. Metaphase
    c. Anaphase
    d. Telophase

27. What is the stage of mitosis in which the chromosomes begin to align?

    a. Prophase
    b. Metaphase
    c. Anaphase
    d. Telophase

28. What is the stage of mitosis in which the paired chromosomes separate, each going to an opposite pole of the cell?

    a. Metaphase
    b. Prophase
    c. Anaphase
    d. Anaphase

29. What is the stage of mitosis in which the two chromosomes are cordoned into new nuclei within the daughter cells?

    a. Metaphase
    b. Prophase
    c. Anaphase
    d. Telophase

30. Squamous, cuboidal and columnar are three kinds of what kind of cell tissue?

    a. Epidermis
    b. Epithelial tissue
    c. Nerve tissue
    d. Muscle tissue

31. What is an important function of epithelial tissue?

    a. Strengthen the muscles
    b. Acting as a protective barrier for the human body
    c. Protect the nerves
    d. Nonexistent. It has no known function

32. What is an important function of connective tissue?

    a. Acting as a protective barrier for the human body
    b. Protect the muscles
    c. Storage of energy
    d. Strengthen the nerves

33. Muscle tissue can _____, bringing out movement and the ability to work.

    a. Divide and conquer
    b. Replicate at will
    c. Relax and contract
    d. Sleep

34. Nervous tissue is specialized to _____

    a. Do work.
    b. Protect the body.
    c. Teach the person to relax.
    d. React to stimuli.

35. Nerve tissue is made up of cells known as _____

    a. Neurons
    b. Protons
    c. Molecules
    d. Atoms

36. The bodily organ system, which protects the person's body from damage, is the _____ system.

    a. Circulatory
    b. Musculoskeletal
    c. Integumentary
    d. Digestive

37. Which of the following are a major part of the integumentary system?

    a. Skeleton
    b. Brain
    c. Skin
    d. Heart

38. What is an example of appendages contained within the integumentary system?

    a. Lungs
    b. Hair and nails
    c. Nostrils
    d. Ears

39. In addition to protecting the body, which of the following is an example of a benefit of the integumentary system?

    a. Circulating blood
    b. Digesting food
    c. Processing information
    d. Regulating temperature

40. How many layers of skin are contained within the human integumentary system (skin)?

    a. One
    b. Two
    c. Three
    d. Four

41. List the three layers of skin.

   a. Proton, neuron, nucleus.
   b. Epidural, Mitochondria, chromosome
   c. Inner, outer, local
   d. Epidermis, dermis and sub dermis.

42. Which sub-layer gives skin its flexibility?

   a. The dermis
   b. Epidermis
   c. Sub dermis
   d. Dermatology

43. What is an example of a minor ailment of the integumentary system?

   a. Skin cancer
   b. Acne
   c. Common cold
   d. Flu

44. Which of the following is an example of a serious ailment of the integumentary system?

   a. Acne
   b. Skin cancer
   c. Heart disease
   d. High blood pressure

45. Which body system is composed mostly of bones?

    a. Respiratory

    b. Endocrine

    c. Musculoskeletal

    d. Integumentary

46. Joints are an example of what within the musculoskeletal system?

    a. Bone tissue

    b. Connective tissue

    c. Muscles

    d. Nerves

47. What is a primary purpose of the musculoskeletal system?

    a. Providing stability to the body.

    b. Distributing blood.

    c. Providing infection control.

    d. Eliminating waste.

48. Another important purpose of the musculoskeletal system is

    a. Moving oxygen.

    b. Cleansing the blood stream.

    c. Relaxing the mind.

    d. Providing form for the body

49. What makes it sometimes difficult to diagnose an ailment within the musculoskeletal system?

    a. Bones resist X-rays.

    b. There are no diseases associated with the musculo-skeletal system.

    c. Its close proximity to other organs within the body.

    d. Its distant proximity away from other organs within the body.

50. What is cartilage?

    a. A flexible, connective tissue that keeps bones from rubbing against each other.

    b. The material that comprises the brain.

    c. A part of human blood responsible for fighting infection.

    d. Another name for the femur.

Section II - Medical Terminology

1. Which, if any, of the following statements is false?

    a. Appendicitis is inflammation of the vermiform appendix.

    b. An appendectomy is a surgical procedure to remove that organ.

    c. Appendicitis may be acute, sub acute, or chronic.

    d. Cathartics or enemas should be administered to prepare the patient for surgery.

2. A/an _____ **is a procedure in which both the** _____ _____ **and some of the surrounding tissue are excised to eliminate cancer or to treat** _____ **or a/an** _____.

 a. A radical prostatectomy is a procedure in which both the prostate gland and some of the surrounding tissue are excised to eliminate cancer or to treat benign prostatic hyperplasia or an enlarged prostate.

 b. A modified prostatectomy is a procedure in which both the prostate gland and some of the surrounding tissue are excised to eliminate cancer or to treat incontinence or an enlarged prostate.

 c. A radical vasectomy is a procedure in which both the prostate gland and some of the surrounding tissue are excised to eliminate cancer or to treat benign prostatic hyperplasia or an enlarged prostate.

 d. A hysterectomy is a procedure in which both the prostate gland and some of the surrounding tissue are excised to eliminate cancer or to treat benign prostatic hyperplasia or an enlarged prostate.

3. The _____ **is a pear-shaped sac located near the right lobe of the liver that holds** _____; **a/an** _____ **is surgery to remove that organ.**

 a. The pancreas is a pear-shaped sac located near the right lobe of the liver that holds bile; a/an pancreatectomy is surgery to remove that organ.

 b. The appendix is a pear-shaped sac located near the right lobe of the liver that holds bile; a/an cholecystectomy is surgery to remove that organ.

 c. The gall bladder is a pear-shaped sac located near the right lobe of the liver that holds bile; a/an appendectomy is surgery to remove that organ.

 d. The gall bladder is a pear-shaped sac located near the right lobe of the liver that holds bile; a/an cholecystectomy is surgery to remove that organ.

4. In cases of bladder stones or the removal of other tissue from the bladder, a/an _____ is performed by the insertion of a thin, lighted instrument through the urethra and into the bladder.

    a. Cystoscopy
    b. Arthroscopy
    c. Laparoscopy
    d. Appendectomy

5. A/an _____ allows a physician to examine the surfaces of the joints and surrounding tissues to diagnose joint complications, repair injuries, remove foreign bodies or monitor disease?

    a. Laminectomy
    b. Dilation
    c. Biopsy
    d. Arthroscopy

6. _____ is the most frequently performed surgery for the treatment of spinal stenosis; the procedure relieves pressure on the spinal cord caused by age-related changes in the spine.

    a. Carpal tunnel surgery
    b. Arthroscopy
    c. Decompressive laminectomy
    d. Lumbar puncture

7. Alternatives for the treatment of breast cancer include either _____ or _____ _____ or a _____ followed by radiation treatment.

   a. Alternatives for the treatment of breast cancer include either simple or modified complete mastectomy or a lumpectomy followed by radiation treatment.

   b. Alternatives for the treatment of breast cancer include either simple or complete mastectomy or a lumpectomy followed by radiation treatment.

   c. Alternatives for the treatment of breast cancer include either simple or radical mastectomy or a biopsy followed by radiation treatment.

   d. Alternatives for the treatment of breast cancer include either simple or modified radical lumpectomy or a mastectomy followed by radiation treatment.

8. Which, if any, of the following statements about bypass surgery is true?

   a. Bypass surgery is frequently performed the patient is experiencing angina.

   b. It is also done in cases of coronary artery disease when plaque has built up in the arteries.

   c. Bypass surgery provide an alternate route for blood flow if a vital artery has become obstructed.

   d. All of the above are true.

9. _____ are a group of tests that are performed together to detect, evaluate, and monitor disease or damage. This procedure determines levels of albumin and bilirubin, among others.

   a. A standard liver panel

   b. A complete blood count

   c. Cerebrospinal fluid analysis

   d. Biopsy

10. A/an _____ refers to the test usually used to screen for HIV infection.

    a. A standard liver panel
    b. Cisternography
    c. Electroencephalography
    d. Enzyme Linked Immunosorbent Assay (ELISA)

11. Which, of any, of the following statements about ultrasound scanning is false?

    a. Ultrasound imaging uses high-frequency sound waves to obtain internal body images.
    b. A neurosonography is an ultrasound of the brain and spinal column that can diagnose strokes and brain tumors.
    c. Ultrasound imaging is less effective than x-rays at revealing soft tissue damage such as torn ligaments, muscles and tendons.
    d. Painful inflammatory processes can be identified through the use of ultrasound imagery.

12. A/an _____ provides information about the number and percentage of red and white blood cells and platelets present. Because abnormally high or low counts are indicative of many types of disease, this test is one of the most commonly performed blood tests in medicine.

    a. Blood culture
    b. Complete blood count (CBC)
    c. Glucose tolerance test
    d. Chorionic villus sampling (CVS)

13. Testing for genetic defects is possible through the use of _____, usually done at 14 to 16 weeks of pregnancy.

    a. Amniocentesis

    b. Chorionic villus sampling (CVS)

    c. Ultrasound imaging

    d. Biopsy

14. Which, if any, of the following statements about neurological examinations are true?

    a. Mental function is determined through mental status exams (MSE) and a global assessment of higher functioning.

    b. Neurological cerebellar testing modalities include dysmetria (finger-to-nose) and ataxia to determine problems with gait.

    c. Examinations are aimed at ruling out the most clinically significant causes and diagnosing the most likely causes.

    d. All of the above are true.

15. Which diagnostic procedure used equipment to develop an image clearly displaying areas of differing density and composition?

    a. Ultrasound imaging

    b. Radiography

    c. Electroencephalography

    d. Fluoroscopy

16. A _____ is a microbiological culture of blood used to detect infections such as bacteria and septicemia.

    a. Complete blood count
    b. Amniocentesis
    c. Blood culture
    d. Chorionic villus sampling (CVS)

17. _____ is a branch of medicine that deals with the _____ system and its production of hormones, which coordinate metabolism, respiration, and excretion, among others. Medical professionals in this field treat persons with diabetes, thyroid diseases, cholesterol disorders, and metabolic disorders.

    a. Endocrinology, endocrine
    b. Gastroenterology, digestive
    c. Hepatology, digestive
    d. Urology

18. Which, if any, of the following statements about geriatrics are false?

    a. Geriatrics is a branch of medicine in which the focus is health care for the aging population.
    b. Geriatrics differs from gerontology, which is the study of the aging process itself.
    c. A geriatrician's practice is limited to persons over the age of 65.
    d. None of the above.

19. _____ is the medical specialty involved in the study of the liver, gallbladder, biliary tree, and pancreas and diseases such as viral hepatitis and alcohol-related conditions.

    a. Hepatology
    b. Immunology
    c. Oncology
    d. Nephrology

20. _____ surgeons use their skills to correct diseases, defects and injuries in the head, neck, face, jaws and the hard and soft tissues of the oral and facial region.

    a. Ear, nose and throat (ENT)
    b. Orthopedic
    c. Reconstructive
    d. Oral and Maxillofacial

21. Which, if any, of the following statements concerning palliative medicine are false?

    a. Palliative medicine is another name for hospice care.

    b. Palliative medicine addresses the needs of patients in all stages of a disease or illness, including those undergoing treatment for curable diseases and those living with chronic illness.

    c. It is a branch of medicine that is focused on both relieving and preventing the suffering of patients.

    d. Palliative medicine relies on input from many sources, including nurses, pharmacists, chaplains and psychologists, among others.

22. Patients who have been diagnosed with acute renal failure, chronic kidney disease, hematuria, kidney stones or hypertension are usually referred to _____.

    a. Pathologists
    b. Hepatologists
    c. Nephrologists
    d. Internists

23. The practice of _____ is concerned with the diagnosis of cancer as well as cancer therapies such as surgery, chemotherapy and radiotherapy as well as follow-up of such cases and palliative care for patients in the terminal stages of cancer.

    a. Pathology
    b. Internal medicine
    c. Oncology
    d. Physical medicine

24. _____ is a branch of medicine that addresses the causes (etiology), mechanisms of development (pathogenesis), structural alterations of cells (morphologic changes), and the consequences of those changes (clinical manifestations or diseases).

    a. Internal medicine
    b. Pathology
    c. Nephrology
    d. None of the above.

Section III – Medical Law and Ethics

1. Which of the following refers to the behaviors the medical professionals with moral integrity are expected to exhibit.

    a. Courtesy
    b. Mores
    c. Customs
    d. Medical ethics

2. The three issues that determine an incident of battery are:

    a. The patient has been given false information about a treatment.
    b. The patient is judged incompetent to consent to treatment and has received improper care.
    c. Care that the patient has refused is forced on them without court authorization.
    d. All of the above

3. The four major principles of medical ethics are:

    a. Autonomy, beneficence, non-malfeasance and justice
    b. Privacy, autonomy, beneficence and justice
    c. Autonomy, beneficence, universality and justice
    d. Autonomy, beneficence, non-malfeasance and morality

4. The definition of a double effect does not state that:

a. A double effect is a byproduct of non-malfeasance

b. The action being considered is in itself either morally good or morally indifferent.

c. There was no direct intention to cause harm.

d. The beneficial result must be disproportionate to the harm caused by the action.

5. Which of these statements about the AMT standards of practice is/are false?

a. Only duly licensed physicians/dentists are required to report any knowledge of professional abuse to the appropriate authorities.

b. As an AMT professional, you must place the welfare of the patient above all other considerations.

c. The judgment of the attending physician/dentist shall be protected and valued, no matter what the circumstances.

d. a) & c)

6. _____ is an ethical principle that states that communication between a patient and a provider must remain private.

a. Autonomy

b. Honesty

c. Consent

d. Confidentiality

7. _____ is the major principle of medical ethics that states that physicians and other medical professionals must act in the best interest of the patient.

    a. Justice
    b. Autonomy
    c. Non-malfeasance
    d. Beneficence

8. The principles of _____ and _____ must be balanced to be certain that any risks involved in medical treatment or procedures is outweighed by the benefit to the patient.

    a. Autonomy and privacy
    b. Dignity and justice
    c. Beneficence and non-malfeasance
    d. Ethics and beneficence

9. _____ is the ethical principle most applicable to the highly publicized issue of universal healthcare.

    a. Justice
    b. Autonomy
    c. Non-malfeasance
    d. Beneficence

10. A _____ system is a process by which treatment is prioritized based on needed personnel and those who are most critically ill or injured.

    a. Disaster
    b. Quarantine
    c. Pandemic
    d. Triage

11. A patient's agreement to treatment based on a clear understanding of their condition and all possible consequences of treatment is a/an _____.

    a. Full disclosure
    b. Legal standard
    c. Logical decision
    d. Informed consent

12. Some exceptions to the rule of informed consent are:

    a. Prior to a common procedure with little risk such as a blood test or in an emergency, life-threatening situation
    b. There are no exceptions to the rule; informed consent must always be obtained prior to treatment.
    c. The patient is a minor.
    d. The patient is suffering advanced dementia.

13. Before a patient exercises their right to refusal of treatment, they must be informed about:

    a. The diagnosis and prognosis of their medical condition
    b. Available alternative treatments and the risks and benefits of those options
    c. The risk and probable outcome of no intervention
    d. All of the above

14. Under certain conditions, a person must submit to _____ treatment, which is medical care or testing without their permission.

    a. Legally mandated
    b. Emergency exception
    c. Life saving
    d. Doctor ordered

15. The situations in which patients must submit to legally mandated treatments include:

   a. The patient has been judged incompetent and has been appointed a guardian.

   b. The patient has been involuntarily confined to a mental institution.

   c. A court has ordered treatment under the authority of public health laws.

   d. All of the above

16. A _____ is an exception to the requirement of informed consent and allows the withholding of information from a patient if such information would cause psychological damage and therefore endanger their physical well-being.

   a. Malpractice suit

   b. Therapeutic exception

   c. Mandated treatment

   d. Autonomy exception

17. Which of the following statements about medical malpractice is false?

   a. Medical malpractice occurs when a negligent act or omission by a doctor or other medical professional results in damage or harm to a patient.

   b. A medical malpractice suit can be filed any time that patient consent was not obtained prior to treatment.

   c. Negligence may involve an error in diagnosis, treatment, or illness management.

   d. A medical malpractice case can also be filed against a hospital for improper care or inadequate training.

18. Which of the following statements about torts is/are false?

   a. Torts are personal civil injuries that reside outside of a contractual relationship.

   b. Torts can be intentional, such as fraud, assault, etc.

   c. Torts result in criminal trials that assess guilt or innocence.

   d. Torts can be unintentional, such as negligence or malpractice.

19. A (n) _____ _____ is a legal document filed in advance by a patient which details their wishes in the event that they are incapacitated.

   a. Last will and testament
   b. Beneficiary list
   c. Advance directive
   d. Funeral plan

20. Which if any of the following statements about living wills is true?

   a. They state the type of care a patient does or does not want to receive at the end of their life.

   b. They are documents in which the patient chooses a surrogate who can make healthcare decisions in the event that they are incapacitated.

   c. They demand that no extraordinary measures such as CPR, are used in an effort to revive the patient.

   d. All of the above.

21. What are the two types of advance directives?

a. A durable power of attorney and a DNR order

b. A funeral plan and a living will

c. A life insurance policy and a durable power of attorney

d. A living will and a durable power of attorney

22. In addition to state laws, _____ is the law that governs the donation of organs and tissues.

a. The Uniform Anatomical Gift Act

b. The Americans with Disabilities Act

c. The Organ Procurement and Use Act

d. There is no law; organ donation is a civil matter between the hospital and a patient's next of kin.

23. While _____ is a mistake or a failure to be careful, _____ includes wrongful conduct by a professional or a failure to meet standards of care that results in harm to another person.

a. While malpractice is a mistake or a failure to be careful, negligence includes wrongful conduct by a professional or a failure to meet standards of care that results in harm to another person.

b. While negligence is a mistake or a failure to be careful, malpractice includes wrongful conduct by a professional or a failure to meet standards of care that results in harm to another person.

c. While substandard behavior is a mistake or a failure to be careful, malpractice includes wrongful conduct by a professional or a failure to meet standards of care that results in harm to another person.

d. While an intentional tort is a mistake or a failure to be careful, malfeasance includes wrongful conduct by a professional or a failure to meet standards of care that results in harm to another person.

24. What conditions usually preclude organ or tissue donation?

    a. Advanced age and metastatic cancer
    b. A history of hepatitis, HIV or AIDS
    c. Sepsis
    d. All of the above

25. In _____, the brain no longer functions organically and the patient is kept alive with a ventilator. When a patient's cerebrum is dead and they are unconscious, cannot think or reason, but may still be breathing, they have experienced _____.

    a. In higher brain death, the brain no longer functions organically and the patient is kept alive with a ventilator. When a patient's cerebrum is dead and they are unconscious, cannot think or reason, but may still be breathing, they have experienced whole brain death.

    b. In whole brain death, the brain no longer functions organically and the patient is kept alive with a ventilator. When a patient's cerebrum is dead and they are unconscious, cannot think or reason, but may still be breathing, they have experienced partial brain death.

    c. In whole brain death, the brain no longer functions organically and the patient is kept alive with a ventilator. When a patient's cerebrum is dead and they are unconscious, cannot think or reason, but may still be breathing, they have experienced higher brain death.

    d. In brain stem death, the brain no longer functions organically and the patient is kept alive with a ventilator. When a patient's cerebrum is dead and they are unconscious, cannot think or reason, but may still be breathing, they have experienced cerebrum brain death.

Section IV – Communication and Patient Education

1. When communicating with another person, _____ is/are used to emphasize an important point, _____ can indicate either great interest or boredom, and _____ can express encouragement or empathy.

    a. When communicating with another person, gestures are used to emphasize an important point, posture can indicate either great interest or boredom, and touch can express encouragement or empathy.

    b. When communicating with another person, touch is used to emphasize an important point, posture can indicate either great interest or boredom, and gestures can express encouragement or empathy.

    c. When communicating with another person, posture is used to emphasize an important point, gestures can indicate either great interest or boredom, and touch can express encouragement or empathy.

    d. When communicating with another person, gestures are used to emphasize an important point, touch can indicate either great interest or boredom, and posture can express encouragement or empathy.

2. A person who is _____ may indicate the desire to place an unconscious barrier between themselves and others.

    a. Avoiding eye contact

    b. Yawning widely

    c. Making wild gestures

    d. Crossing their arms across their chest

3. Which, if any, of the following statements about eye contact are false?

   a. Consistent eye contact can indicate a positive reaction to a speaker.

   b. Consistent eye contact can indicate a lack of trust in the speaker.

   c. The use of eye contact may be dependent on the culture of the listener.

   d. None of these statements are false.

4. _____ is a technique used to put people at ease.

   a. Speaking softly
   b. Making eye contact
   c. Mirroring body language
   d. Leaning forward

5. Which, if any, of these statements about body language are false?

   a. Everyone uses some form of body language to communicate.

   b. Interpretations of body language are universal to all cultures.

   c. The study of body language is called kinetic interpretation.

   d. Indications of emotion such as smiling when happy are universal.

6. _____ can signal a lack of interest or an unfriendly attitude and can make therapeutic communication difficult to achieve.

    a. Eye contact
    b. Questioning
    c. Empathy
    d. Nonverbal communication

7. If a patient asks a question that is beyond the scope of your practice, the best response would be to:

    a. Make your best guess based on what you know.
    b. Tell the patient that you will find them the correct answer.
    c. Change the subject.
    d. Give them a book on the subject.

8. _____ is an important communication technique in which phrases such as "go on," please continue," and "tell me more" are used to encourage the patient.

    a. Facilitation
    b. Amplification
    c. Reflection
    d. Mirroring

9. _____ involves repeating something the patient just said to gain more specific information and to show that you are paying attention.

    a. Facilitation
    b. Reflection
    c. Mirroring
    d. None of the above

10. What are the two goals of the technique of summarization?

    a. To ensure that the information that you've collected is accurate and complete and to signal the end of the interview

    b. To obtain more specific information and to show that you are paying attention

    c. To gain the patient's trust and to obtain more specific information

    d. To make the interview as short as possible and to follow the rules as determined by the HMO.

11. _____ is restating something that a patient has said, usually in fewer words and with emphasis on the main points of their statement.

    a. Attending

    b. Paraphrasing

    c. Clarifying

    d. Perception checking

12. When _____ is used in active listening, it demonstrates that you understand the patient's experience and allows them to evaluate their feeling by hearing them expressed by someone else.

    a. Paraphrasing

    b. Summarization

    c. Clarifying

    d. Primary empathy

13. The steps to attentive listening include:

a. Maintaining eye contact and facing the person squarely

b. Sitting up straight and maintaining eye contact

c. Taking careful notes and leaning toward the speaker

d. Relaxing in your seat and slightly averting your eyes

14. Facial expression, posture and tone of voice are elements of _____.

a. Open-ended questions

b. Nonverbal communication

c. Orientation process

d. Good manners

15. Which, if any, of the following statements about nonverbal communication are true?

a. Nonverbal communications are less reliable that verbal communication

b. Nonverbal communications remain the same, regardless of ethnicity or culture.

c. Nonverbal communications always send a clear message.

d. Nonverbal communications can emphasize or contradict verbal messages.

16. _____ is/are used to obtain the most complete information available.

a. Questionnaires and surveys

b. Admission forms

c. Open-ended questions

d. Interviews

17. Which, if any, of the following statements is false?

   a. An interviewer should never ask close-ended questions.

   b. A close-ended question is one that can be answered "yes" or "no."

   c. An example of a close-ended question would be "Have you been having headaches for a long time?"

   d. A close-ended question can be used to verify information already obtained.

18. _____ provides encourages the patient to continue talking without indicating agreement or disagreement.

   a. Smiling

   b. Leaning forward

   c. Nodding

   d. Paraphrasing

19. Using phrases that address a person's feelings, such as "You must be worried about your headaches," demonstrates _____.

   a. Empathy

   b. Interest

   c. Acceptance

   d. Recognition

20. _____ can be an effective way to communicate with children.

   a. Telling stories

   b. Reading books

   c. Watching cartoons

   d. Role playing

Part II – Administrative Medical Assisting

Section I – Insurance

1. What type of Medical Insurance plan does the employer typically pay?

    a. Health Maintenance Organization (HMO)
    b. Indemnity
    c. Major Medical
    d. None of the Above

2. Preferred Provider Organization (PPO) insurance:

    a. is a list of health care providers that provided services at a discounted rate.
    b. does not cover primary care.
    c. usually has deductibles and limits.
    d. does not offer a discounted rate.

3. Which program offers health care to dependents and spouses of service women and men?

    a. Medigap
    b. Tricare
    c. Commercial Insurance
    d. CHAMPVA

4. What Medical plan is for people over 65?

    a. Medicaid
    b. Tricare
    c. CHAMPVA
    d. Medicare

5. What is an RVU?

    a. the system for reimbursement.
    b. a component that is multiplied by a monetary conversion factor to calculate physicians costs.
    c. a list of procedures.
    d. a list of procedures and their cost.

6. What is the insured person's child called?

    a. coinsured
    b. dependent
    c. group insured member
    d. family insured member

7. What is the 'point of service?'

    a. The place where they bought the insurance.
    b. The place where the patient was injured.
    c. The place where the service is delivered.
    d. The place where they pay for the service.

8. What is pre-certification?

    a. getting approval for a service or procedure
    b. determining if the service is covered
    c. determining the amount the insurance company will cover
    d. None of the Above

9. What type of insurance covers significant illness?

a. Medicare
b. Major Medical
c. Indemnity
d. HMO

10. Medicare Part A covers

a. hospital inpatient costs
b. hospital outpatient costs
c. No hospital costs
d. Doctor office visits

11. Medicare Part B covers

a. physician costs
b. outpatient services
c. physician costs
d. physician costs

12. Which of the following are NOT eligible for TRICARE:

a. Veterans
b. Army service men and women
c. Special Forces men and women
d. Spouses of service men or women convicted of spousal or child abuse

13. Which of the following is NOT a benefit under Worker's Compensation?

a. Prostheses
b. Spousal treatment
c. Death Benefits to Survivors
d. Permanent disability payments

14. Which of the following methods of insurance payment is based on a relative value system?

   a. Fee Schedule
   b. RBRVS
   c. UCR
   d. Capitation

Section II – Coding and Claims

15. What level of HCPCS covers new procedures not given a permanent CPT code?

   a. Level I
   b. Level II
   c. Level III
   d. None of the Above

16. What Level of HCPCS covers codes not covered by CPT codes?

   a. Level I
   b. Level II
   c. Level III
   d. None of the Above

17. What Level of HCPCS covers ambulance services?

   a. Level I
   b. Level II
   c. Level III
   d. None of the Above

18. What Level of HCPCS covers pharmaceuticals?

a. Level I
b. Level II
c. Level III
d. None of the Above

19. What level of HCPCS covers regionally approved Medicare procedures?

a. Level I
b. Level II
c. Level III
d. None of the Above

20. Which Procedural Code has five numbers?

a. CPT or HCPCS Level I
b. HCPCS Level II
c. HCPCS Level III
d. None of the Above

21. What Procedural Code has Letters from A - V and 4 numbers?

a. CPT or HCPCS Level I
b. HCPCS Level II
c. HCPCS Level III
d. None of the Above

22. The HCPCS Level II code for Orthotic/Prosthetic procedures is:

a. P-codes
b. G-codes
c. A-codes
d. L-codes

23. The HCPCS Level II code for Durable Medical Equipment is:

   a. G-codes
   b. L-codes
   c. E-codes
   d. M-codes

24. What Procedural Codes have Letters W - A and 4 numbers?

   a. CPT or HCPCS Level I
   b. HCPCS Level II
   c. HCPCS Level III
   d. None of the Above

Section III – Finance and Bookkeeping

25. What is included on the Day Sheet?

   a. Charges and payments received
   b. Patients and doctors names
   c. Itemized statement of a patient's accounts receivable
   d. List of all monies owed

26. What type of account is the Day Sheet?

   a. Accounts Payable
   b. General Ledger
   c. Accounts Receivable
   d. Patient Ledger

27. A medical office has run out of pencils and paper. How should you purchase these?

    a. With a company check.

    b. With petty cash.

    c. With your own funds and ask for reimbursement.

    d. With cash from the cash box.

28. All funds owed for items such as rent are:

    a. Accounts Receivable

    b. Accounts Payable

    c. Receipts

    d. General Ledger items

29. What form would a courier issue to the office upon receipt of a package?

    a. Invoice

    b. Receipt

    c. Bill of Lading

    d. Purchase Order

30. Funds owed to a physician from patients and others are called

    a. Account Receivable

    b. Account Payable

    c. Net Income

    d. Expenses

31. What form has all the information for a patient to file an insurance claim?

    a. Superbill

    b. Invoice

    c. Receipt

    d. Ledger

32. A Debit to an account:

   a. is an amount owed.
   b. is an amount paid.

33. The amount of income a physician's office makes after taxes and expenses is:

   a. Gross Income
   b. Wage
   c. Gross expenses
   d. Net income

34. Comparing the check book to the bank statement is called

   a. Auditing
   b. Reconciliation
   c. Balancing
   d. Account balancing

Part III – Clinical Medical Assisting
Section I – Asepsis

1. Which type of Asepsis eliminates all microorganisms?

   a. Medical Asepsis
   b. Surgical Asepsis
   c. All asepsis
   d. None of the Above

2. Which method of Asepsis allows lotion to be applied?

   a. Medical Asepsis
   b. Surgical Asepsis
   c. No asepsis method allows lotion to be applied
   d. All asepsis methods allow lotion to be applied

3. Which method of asepsis requires hands to be held downwards while rinsing?

   a. Medical Asepsis
   b. Surgical Asepsis
   c. All asepsis methods
   d. No asepsis methods

4. The chain of infection requires a means of transmission. Which of the following is NOT a means of transmission?

   a. Dirty hands
   b. Air
   c. Contaminated food
   d. Sneezing

5. The primary reason for aseptic procedures is to

   a. Protect patients
   b. Protect patients and health care providers
   c. Wipe out all bacteria in the office
   d. None of the above

6. The correct setting for an autoclave is:

   a. 2000 F for a least 40 minutes
   b. 2540 F for 15 minutes
   c. 2500 F for at least 20 minutes
   d. 4000 F for 10 minutes

7. What is the recommended method of turning off a hand faucet after washing your hands?

   a. After applying lotion
   b. With a paper or cloth towel
   c. After putting on surgical gloves
   d. None of the Above

Section II - Vital Signs and Physical Modalities

8. Which of the following is not a vital sign?

   a. Blood pressure
   b. Body temperature
   c. Psychological state
   d. Respiration

9. What is a normal oral temperature?

a. 98.6 F or 37 C
b. 37 F or 98.6 C
c. 96.8 F or 37 F
d. 99.6 F or 38 C

10. What is a normal aural temperature?

a. 96.8 F or 37 C
b. 98.6 F or 37 C
c. 99.6 F or 38 C
d. 97.6 F or 37 C

11. Which therapy is used in the initial phase of treatment?

a. Thermotherapy
b. Cryotherapy
c. Hydrotherapy
d. None of the Above

12. Which therapy causes vasodilation?

a. Cryotherapy
b. Hydrotherapy
c. Thermotherapy
d. All of the above

13. What is physiatry?

a. A treatment that reduces pain and swelling by improving circulation
b. A treatment that causes blood vessels to constrict
c. The diagnosis and treatment of disease using physical means
d. None of the above

14. What type of therapy causes blood vessels to constrict (vasoconstriction)?

    a. Cryotherapy
    b. Hydrotherapy
    c. Therotherapy
    d. None of the Above

15. What are isometric exercises?

    a. Exercises that expand opposing muscles without shortening
    b. Exercises that contract opposing muscles without shortening
    c. Exercises performed on the patient
    d. None of the above

16. What are resistance exercises?

    a. Exercises that contract opposing muscles
    b. Exercises with counter-pressure
    c. Exercises that expand opposing muscles
    d. None of the above

17. What type of exam evaluates the extent of movement of a patient's arm?

    a. Manipulation
    b. Traction
    c. Range of motion
    d. None of the Above

18. What type of exercise would you recommend when the patient is unable to move the body part?

   a. Passive exercise
   b. Isometric exercise
   c. Manipulation
   d. Resistance exercise

Section III – Clinical Pharmacology

19. What is the difference between a Schedule IV and Schedule V drug?

   a. Schedule IV requires a prescription and Schedule V does not.
   b. Schedule V requires a prescription and Schedule IV does not.
   c. Schedule IV has moderate potential for abuse and Schedule V has low potential.
   d. Schedule V has moderate potential for abuse and Schedule IV has low potential.

20. What is the difference between Schedule II and Schedule III drugs?

   a. Schedule II drugs have a high potential for abuse and Schedule III drugs have a moderate potential for abuse
   b. Schedule III drugs have a high potential for abuse and Schedule II drugs have a moderate potential for abuse

21. Which of the following is a Schedule II drug?

   a. Valium
   b. Heroin
   c. Barbiturates
   d. Cocaine

22. What is a common antidiarrheal drug?

    a. Lidocaine
    b. Lomotil
    c. Mylanta
    d. Benadryl

23. What is the common use of Antiemetic drugs?

    a. Relief of fever
    b. Relief of nausea
    c. Decreases depression
    d. Controls high blood pressure

Section IV – Minor Surgery

24. Identify the instrument below:

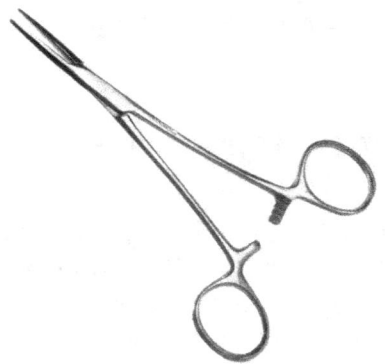

    a. Hemostats
    b. Tenaculum
    c. Suture removal scissors
    d. None of the Above

25. Identify the instrument below:

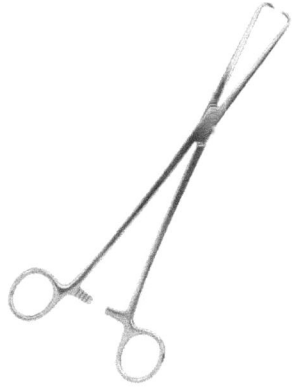

   a. Hemostats
   b. Tenaculum
   c. Surgical scissors
   d. Bandage scissors

26. Identify the instrument below:

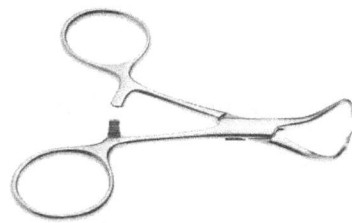

   a. Hemostats
   b. Towel Clip
   c. Surgical scissors
   d. Bandage scissors

27. Identify the instrument below:

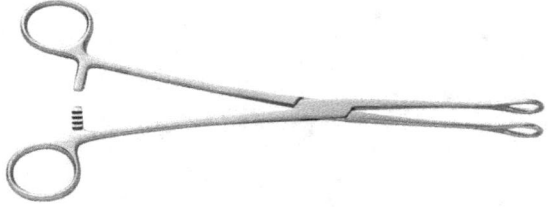

    a. Ring Forceps
    b. Suture removal scissors
    c. Tenaculum
    d. Hemostats

28. How should hands be rinsed during surgical hand washing?

    a. Rinse hands in a downward position.
    b. Rinse hands in an upward position.
    c. Rinse hands flat.
    d. No specification.

29. What is the proper procedure for applying local anaesthetic?

    a. Show the physician the label
    b. Hold the vial upside down.
    c. Pass the vial to the physician.
    d. None of the Above.

Section V – Lab and ECG

30. What is the adult normal range bleeding time?

    a. 2 - 9 minutes
    b. 5 - 10 minutes
    c. 1 - 5 minutes
    d. 7 - 15 minutes

31. What is the adult normal range for cholesterol (total)?

    a. 90- 100 mEq/L
    b. 80 - 95 mEq/L
    c. 98 - 110 mEq/L
    d. 95 - 120 mEq/L

32. What is an adult normal range reading for glucose?

    a. 80-110 mg/dL
    b. 100 - 120 mg/dL
    c. 75 - 95 mg/dL
    d. 110 - 130 mg/dL

33. What is a normal result for a glucose reagent strip urinalysis?

    a. Dark Yellow
    b. Light Pink
    c. Negative
    d. Positive

34. What is a normal result for a pH reagent strip urinalysis?

    a. 4.5 - 8
    b. 5.5 - 10
    c. 7 - 10.5
    d. None of the Above.

35. What is a normal range for hemoglobin (Hb)?

    a. 5.2 - 11.7 g/dL
    b. 15.5 - 20.4 g/dL
    c. 14.7 - 19.5 g/dL
    d. 11.7 - 16.0 g/dL

36. What component is approximately 55% of the whole blood?

    a. Red blood cells
    b. Plasma
    c. Serum
    d. Buffy coat

37. What component is located at the bottom of the specimen tube?

    a. Red blood cells
    b. Plasma
    c. Buffy coat
    d. Serum

38. What is a collection tube with a grey top used for?

    a. Blood for glucose and alcohol testing

    b. Blood for urgent chemical tests

    c. Blood for hematology testing

    d. Serum for chemistry and serology

39. What is the Atrial Systole phase of the cardiac cycle?

    a. Contraction of atria

    b. Relaxation of the ventricles

    c. Relaxation of atria

    d. Contraction of ventricles

40. Which of the following describes the ventricle systole phase of the cardiac cycle?

    a. Contraction of atria

    b. Contraction of the ventricles

    c. Relaxation of atria

    d. Relaxation of the ventricles

41. Which of the following describes the Atrial Diastole phase of the cardiac cycle?

    a. Contraction of atria

    b. Relaxation of atrial

    c. Contraction of the ventricles

    d. Relaxation of the ventricles

42. Identify the segment and interval labelled 1 and 2 below:

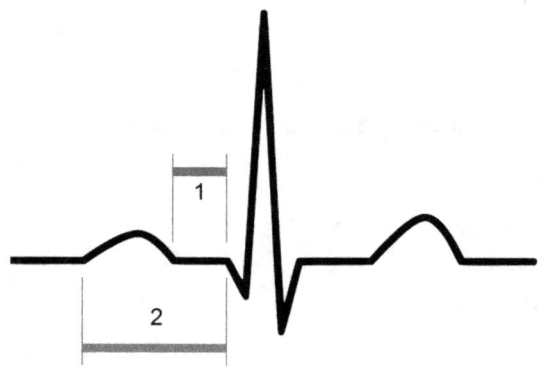

a. 1 is the PR interval and 2 is the PR segment
b. 1 is the PR segment and 2 is the PR interval
c. 1 is the ST cycle and 2 is the ST segment
d. 1 is the ST segment and 2 is the ST cycle

43. Identify the red line is the diagram below:

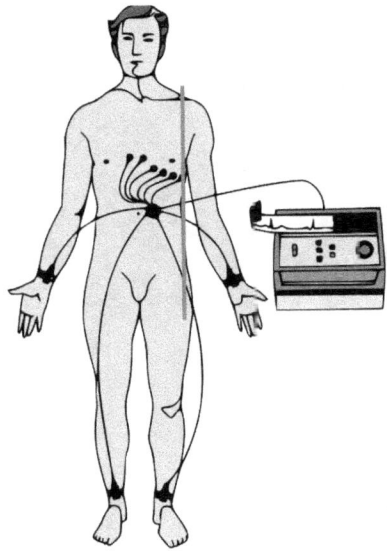

a. Midclavicular line
b. Anterior axillary line
c. Midaxillary line
d. Horizontal plan of V4-V6

44. Identify the region marked 1 on the diagram below:

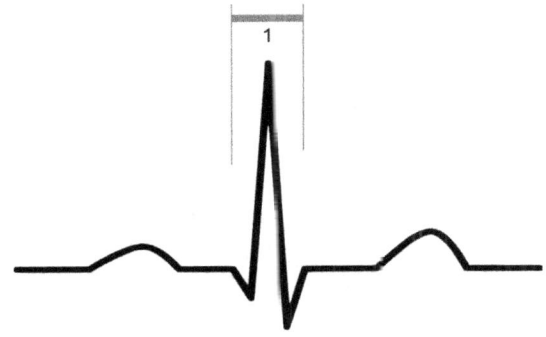

a. QRS interval
b. PR interval
c. ST interval
d. QT interval

45. Identify the red line in the diagram below:

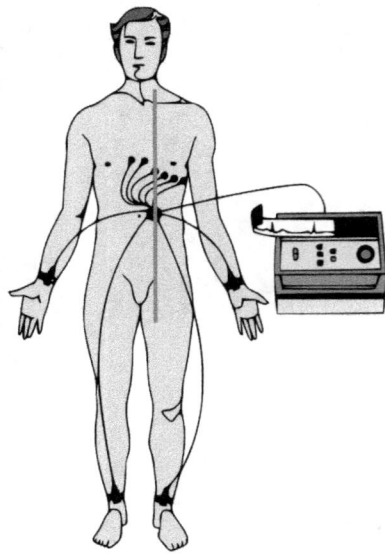

a. Anterior auxiliary line
b. Midclavicular line
c. Midaxillary line
d. Horizontal plane of V4-V6

Answer Key

Part 1 – General Medical Assisting Knowledge

Section I – Anatomy and Physiology

1. C
The abdomen can be divided by two lines into 4 quadrants or by 4 lines into 9 regions.

The two lines that divide the abdomen into quadrants form a cross, the centre of which is positioned over the umbilicus (belly button). These quadrants are often used to indicate the location of pain.

2. A
The Left upper quadrant of the abdomen, is often abbreviated as LUQ, contains the stomach, spleen, left lobe of the liver, body of the pancreas, left kidney and adrenal gland.

3. D
The right upper quadrant of the abdomen, often abbreviated as RUQ, contains the liver, gall bladder, duodenum and had of the pancreas.

4. A
The Right lower quadrant of the human abdomen, often abbreviated as RLQ, contains the appendix and ascending colon.

5. B
Medical personnel divide the abdomen into smaller regions to facilitate study and discussion.

6. A
The stomach and colon are both in the Left Upper Quadrant, together with, liver, spleen, left kidney, pancreas and large intestine.

7. C
The commonly used abbreviations for the Quadrants are, Right Upper Quadrant, RUQ, Left Upper Quadrant, LUQ, Right Lower Quadrant, RLQ, Left Lower Quadrant, LLQ.

8. D
All of the above. The Large Intestine passes through all of the quadrants.

9. B
The stomach and colon are both in the Left Upper Quadrant, together with, liver, spleen, left kidney, pancreas and large intestine.

10. A
The gallbladder is located in the Right Upper Quadrant together with the liver, right kidney, colon, pancreas and large intestine.

11. D
There are many complex interactions that take place inside of the human body. These processes make sure that the internal balance is always within a range that is normal and healthy. The kidneys, for instance, are responsible for re-absorption of substances in the blood, keeping blood sugar levels regulated, and keeping the levels of salt and iron within the normal range, managing blood ph levels, and controlling the excretion of wastes such as urea.

12. A
Homeostasis is the property of a system that regulates its internal environment and tends to maintain a stable, constant condition of properties like temperature or pH.

13. D
The amount of energy / calories that your body requires to maintain itself is metabolism.

14. B
Exercise and low fat diets will increase metabolism. Choice B, a man who is past 30 and whose body is losing muscle is the only choice.

Practice Test Questions Set 1   73

15. A
Exercise will increase metabolism, so aerobic exercise.

16. A
The kidneys are responsible for regulating fluid balance.

17. B
Fluid balance is important, because water comprises about 60-70% of a person's weight.

18. B
Metabolism slows with aging.

19. D
"Met" refers to the person's metabolic rate.

20. A
Fluid balance is important, because the human body loses water every day through urination, perspiration, feces, and breathing.

21. D
The smallest unit of life in our bodies is the cell.

22. B
The interior of cells are separated from the exterior environment by the biological membranes known as plasma membranes or cell membranes. This membrane controls the flow of substances in and out of the cells by being selectively permeable to organic molecules and ions.

23. A
Cell division is the process by which a parent cell divides into two or more daughter cells. Cell division is usually a small segment of a larger cell cycle.

24. C
Mitosis is the process by which a eukaryotic cell separates the chromosomes in its cell nucleus into two identical sets in two separate nuclei. The process of mitosis is fast and highly complex. The sequence of events is divided into stages corresponding to the completion of one set of activities and the start of the next. These stages are interphase, prophase,

prometaphase, metaphase, anaphase and telophase.

25. B
Mitosis is the process by which a eukaryotic cell separates the chromosomes in its cell nucleus into two identical sets in two separate nuclei. [1]

26. A
Prophase, is a stage of mitosis in which the chromatin condenses (it becomes shorter and fatter) into a highly ordered structure called a chromosome in which the chromatin becomes visible.

27. B
In the eukaryotic cell cycle there is a mitosis stage known as the metaphase, which is when highly coiled, condensed chromosomes, that carry genetic information, line up with the cell's center and are then split between the daughter cells. The prometaphase prepares for this stage and the anaphase continues the process, while the metaphase itself involves microtubles, which were formed in the prophase, attaching themselves to the kinetochores that they find.

28. D
Anaphase is the stage of mitosis or meiosis hen chromosomes move to opposite poles of the cell. The anaphase starts when the metaphase-to-anaphase transition begins the process of regulating triggering. The destruction of cyclin, which is essential to the metaphase, marks the beginning of the transition. Anaphase, on the other hand, starts with the cleavage of securin, which is important to inhibiting the separase protease. The separase then cleaves the protein that holds chromatids together, known as cohesin.

29. D
Telophase is a stage in both meiosis and mitosis in a eukaryotic cell. This stage of the cell's life reverses the events of both prophase and prometaphase. Here, two daughter nuclei will form inside of the cell. The daughter cells' nuclear envelope forms out of the parent cells' nuclear envelopes. The nuclei reappears when both chromatid pair has a nuclear envelope formed round it.

30. B
Epithelium is one of the four basic types of animal tissue, along with the connective tissue, muscle tissue, and nervous tissue. The cavities and surfaces of different body structures are lined with epithelial tissue, which also forms many of the body's glands. These cells can function as a part of selective absorption, secretion, transcellular transport, detection of sensation, and protection.

To classify the simple epithelial tissues, shape is normally the standard. The four classes used for classification are: 1) Simple Squamous 2) Simple Cuboidal 3) Simple Columnar and 4) Pseudostratified

31. B
Epithelial tissue acts as a protective barrier for the human body.

32. C
The functions of connective tissue are, storage of energy, protection of organs, providing structural framework for the body and connection of body tissues.

33. C
Muscle tissue has the ability to relax and contract, bringing out movement and the ability to work.

34. D
Nervous tissue is specialized to react to stimuli.

35. A
Nerve tissue is made of cells called neurons.

36. C
The integumentary system is the organ system that protects the body from damage, comprising the skin and its appendages, including hair, scales, feathers, and nails.

37. C
The integumentary system comprises the skin and its various appendages, including hair, scales, feathers, and nails.

38. B
The appendages of the integumentary system are hair, scales, feathers, and nails.

39. D
The integumentary system has a variety of functions; it may serve to waterproof, cushion, and protect the deeper tissues, excrete wastes, and regulate temperature, and is the attachment site for sensory receptors to detect pain, sensation, pressure, and temperature.

40. C
The human skin (integumentary) is composed of a minimum of 3 major layers of tissue, the Epidermis, the Dermis and Hypodermis.

41. D
The human skin (integumentary) is composed of a minimum of 3 major layers of tissue, the Epidermis, the Dermis and Hypodermis. [2]

42. A
The middle layer of skin, known as the dermis, is constructed in a diffusely bundled and woven pattern using dense connective tissues such as elastin and collagen. These dermis layers are designed to provide the integument with elasticity and allow the tissue to flex and stretch, while remaining resistant against sagging, distorting, or wrinkling.

43. B
Acne is an example of a minor ailment of the integumentary system.

44. B
Skin cancer is an example of a serious ailment of the integumentary system.

45. C
Musculoskeletal is a body system comprised mostly of the bones.

46. B
Joints are an example of connective tissue within the mus-

culoskeletal system.

47. A
One of the primary purposes of the musculoskeletal system is providing stability to the body.

48. D
Another primary purpose of the musculoskeletal system is providing form for the body.

49. C
It is difficult to diagnose an ailment within the musculoskeletal system because of its close proximity to other organs.

50. A
The joints between bones, the ear, the elbow, the rib cage, the knee, the ankle, the intervertebral discs, and the bronchial tubes are all constructed out of the flexible connective tissue called cartilage. It is found in humans and animals, as well, and is stiffer and less flexible than muscle tissue, while being softer and less rigid that bones.

Section II – Medical Terminology

1. D
Enemas are never administered to prepare patients for surgery.

2. A
A radical prostatectomy is a procedure in which both the prostate gland and some of the surrounding tissue are excised to eliminate cancer or to treat benign prostatic hyperplasia or an enlarged prostate.

3. D
The gall bladder is a pear-shaped sac located near the right lobe of the liver that holds bile; a/an cholecystectomy is surgery to remove that organ.

4. A
In cases of bladder stones or the removal of other tissue from the bladder, a/an Cystoscopy is performed by the insertion of a thin, lighted instrument through the urethra and into the bladder.

5. D
A/an Arthroscopy allows a physician to examine the surfaces of the joints and surrounding tissues to diagnose joint complications, repair injuries, remove foreign bodies or monitor disease.

6. C
Decompressive laminectomy is the most frequently performed surgery for the treatment of spinal stenosis; the procedure relieves pressure on the spinal cord caused by age-related changes in the spine.

7. D
Alternatives for the treatment of breast cancer include either simple or modified radical lumpectomy or a mastectomy followed by radiation treatment.

8. D
Bodily organs can sometimes adhere to the peritoneum, a two-layered membrane lining the abdominal cavity and covering abdominal organs; when this occurs, it the problem is corrected through surgical release of peritoneal adhesions.

9. A
A standard liver panel are a group of tests that are performed together to detect, evaluate, and monitor disease or damage. This procedure determines levels of albumin and bilirubin, among others.

10. D
A/an Enzyme Linked Immunosorbent Assay (ELISA) refers to the test usually used to screen for HIV infection.

11. C
The following statement is false: Ultrasound imaging is less effective than x-rays at revealing soft tissue damage such as torn ligaments, muscles and tendons.

12. B
A/an complete blood count (CBC) provides information about the number and percentage of red and white blood cells and platelets present. Because abnormally high or low counts are indicative of many types of disease, this test is one of the most commonly performed blood tests in medicine.

13. A
Testing for genetic defects is possible through the use of amniocentesis, usually done at 14 to 16 weeks of pregnancy.

14. D
All of the statements are true.

15. B
Radiography diagnostic procedure used equipment to develop an image clearly displaying areas of differing density and composition.

16. C
A blood culture is a microbiological culture of blood used to detect infections such as bacteria and septicemia.

17. A
Endocrinology is a branch of medicine that deals with the endocrine system and its production of hormones, which coordinate metabolism, respiration, and excretion, among others. Medical professionals in this field treat persons with diabetes, thyroid diseases, cholesterol disorders, and metabolic disorders.

18. C
A geriatrician's practice is limited to persons over the age of 65 is false. This sub-specialty of internal and family medicine focuses specifically on the hare of elderly people. The goal is to treat and prevent disabilities and diseases in older people to promote their good health. No specific age has been set as to when a patient can see a geriatrician, however. The decision is normally made by assessing the individual patient's needs and the specialists that are available.

19. A
Hepatology is the medical specialty involved in the study of the liver, gallbladder, biliary tree, pancreas and diseases such as viral hepatitis and alcohol-related conditions.

20. D
Oral and Maxillofacial surgeons use their skills to correct diseases, defects and injuries in the head, neck, face, jaws and the hard and soft tissues of the oral and facial region.

21. A
Palliative medicine is another name for hospice care is false. Palliative care specializes in the area of dealing with suffering patients and preventing and relieving their ailments. This is different from hospice care in that it is well suited for any stage of a patient's disease, including both the treatment of curable illnesses and those who live with chronic diseases, as well as end of life treatment for fatal ailments. Using an approach that is multidisciplinary, palliative medicine relies on information from nurses, chaplains, physicians, pharmacists, psychologists, social workers, and a variety of other healthcare professionals to create a plan of care that caters to every part of a person's life.

22. C
Kidney diseases are diagnosed and treated under the specialty of nephrology. This can involve hypertension, electrolyte disturbances, and other diseases, while caring for patients who need renal replacement therapy, such as renal transplants and dialysis.

23. C
Oncology is a branch of medicine that deals with cancer. Someone who practices oncology as a medical professional is an oncologist.

Oncology deals with:

- Diagnosing any kind of cancer
- Cancer therapy like surgery, radiotherapy, chemotherapy, and others
- Follow-up appointments after a patient's successful treatment

- Continued palliative care for those with terminal malignancies
- Cancer care concerns with ethical questions
- Efforts to screen populations of people, or relatives of patients when dealing with hereditary cancers like breast cancer [3]

24. B
Pathology is the precise study and diagnosis of disease. There are four components of disease that pathology concerns itself with: cause (or etiology), the mechanism of development (or pathogenesis), alterations to the structure of the cells (morphologic changes), and what consequences those changes have (clinical manifestations).

Further than this, pathology is divided into categories based on either the system that is being studied (veterinary pathology and animal disease) or what the focus of the study is on (forensic pathology and cause of death determinations).

Section III – Medical Law and Ethics

1. D
The system of moral principles that practitioners apply to their values and judgements are known as medical ethics. When studied as a scholarly pursuit, this is the study of not only practical applications in medical treatment, but the history of the practice, as well as the sociological, theological, and philosophical aspects.

2. D
All the statements are true.
The patient was given fake information about the treatments
The patient has not only received improper care, but has been judged unable to consent to the treatment
The care was refused by the patient, but forced on them without being authorized by a court

Battery is specifically the unlawful use of physical contact. This is different from the criminal offence of assault, which is the threat or fear of that contact.

In The United States, simple battery is defined as using force against another person, with offensive or harmful contact being the end result. The term is used in a general way to describe any unlawful physical contact, although the law itself is more specific. In particular, battery is defined as "any unlawful touching of the person of another by the aggressor himself, or by a substance put in motion by him." In the majority of battery cases, it is subject to statutes and can change in severity depending on each jurisdiction.

3. A
The four major principles of medical ethics are autonomy, beneficence, non-malfeasance and justice.

Autonomy: The patient can refuse their treatment, or choose a course of action
Beneficence: The doctor should always act in the patient's best interest
Non-malfeasance: "First, do no harm"
Justice: Scarce resources must be distributed according to who needs what kind of treatment and what would be fair

These are not answers to handling situations, but they are a framework for understanding the conflicts that can arise.

4. B
Double effect does not state that, the action being considered is in itself either morally good or morally indifferent.

Double effect, known as the principle of double effect, the doctrine of double effect, or the rule of double effect is often abbreviated as DDE or PDE. This is the ethical criteria that is used to evaluate the decisions a practitioner should make when the legitimate act could also result in a harmful effect that would usually be avoided.

The criteria states that an action that has known harmful effects can be justified if it fits a number of criteria:

- The nature of the action must be good, or at the very least neutral morally

- The procedure must have a good effect that is intentional and is the ends, not the means
- The circumstances must justify the action and the bad effects must be outweighed by the good results

5. D
The following statements about the AMT standards of practice are false:

- Only duly licensed physicians/dentists are required to report any knowledge of professional abuse to the appropriate authorities.
- The judgment of the attending physician/dentist shall be protected and valued, no matter what the circumstances.

6. D
Confidentiality is an ethical principle that states that communication between a patient and a provider must remain private.

7. D
Beneficence is the major principle of medical ethics that states that physicians and other medical professionals must act in the best interest of the patient.

Actions that are meant to enhance others' wellbeing are referred to with the phrase beneficence. When it comes to the medical world, this specifically refers to actions with the best interests of each patient in mind. The problem comes from the lack of a definition of the practices that help patients in the best way.

8. A
The principles of autonomy and privacy must be balanced to be certain that any risks involved in medical treatment or procedures is outweighed by the benefit to the patient.

9. A
Justice concerns the distribution of scarce health resources, and the decision of who gets what treatment (fairness and equality). [4]

10. D
A triage system is a process by which treatment is prioritized based on needed personnel and those who are most critically ill or injured.

Assessing the severity of a patient's condition in order to determine their priority is known as triage. At a time when resources are scarce, this helps to ration the treatments in order to provide the best care. There are two categories of triage: advanced triage and simple triage. This can be used to decide the order of emergency treatments, the order of emergency patient transportation, or the destination of the patient for treatment. This triage process is done when patients first arrive at an emergency facility, when they are phoning in emergency calls, or any other time that a patient has an emergency that must be assessed.

11. D
In legal terms, informed consent refers to the consent that a patient gives when they have met the minimum standards for consenting to a procedure. Unless there is fraud potentially taking place, this is usually redundant. A patient can be said to give informed consent when they clearly understand all of the facts, consequences, and implications of an action and can clearly appreciate the situation. For a patient to be able to do this, the patient must have the ability to reason and have knowledge of all of the relevant facts when they give consent to a medical professional. Any impaired reasoning faculties or impaired judgement that make a patient incapable of giving informed consent can include things such as basic emotional or intellectual immaturity, high stress levels or conditions such as mental retardation or PTSD, severe mental illness, extreme lack of sleep, late stage Alzheimer's disease, or remaining in a coma.

12. A
Prior to a common procedure with little risk such as a blood test or in an emergency, life-threatening situation are exceptions to the rule of informed consent.

13. D
Before a patient exercises their right to refusal of treatment, they must be informed about:

- The diagnosis and prognosis of their medical condition
- Available alternative treatments and the risks and benefits of those options
- The risk and probable outcome of no intervention

14. A
Legally mandated treatment is medical care or testing without their permission.

15. D
The situations in which patients must submit to legally mandated treatments include:

- The patient has been judged incompetent and has been appointed a guardian.
- The patient has been involuntarily confined to a mental institution.
- A court has ordered treatment under the authority of public health laws.

16. B
A therapeutic exception is an exception to the requirement of informed consent and allows the withholding of information from a patient if such information would cause psychological damage and therefore endanger their physical well-being.

17. B
The following statement about medical malpractice is false, a medical malpractice suit can be filed any time that patient consent was not obtained prior to treatment.

The problem of medical malpractice is defined as negligence by medical professionals. That can be either omission or action taken by a healthcare professional where the provided treatment fails to meet the standard of practice that is accepted and set by the medical community, causing death or severe injury as a direct result, many times due to medical errors by a party involved. The standards and regulations for medical malpractice can vary by country and jurisdiction within counties. To protect themselves, health care providers are able to purchase professional liability insurance, which helps offset costs of medical malpractice lawsuits.

18. C
Torts result in criminal trials that assess guilt or innocence is false.

In common law jurisdictions, tort is a wrong act that breaches civil duties that are owed to another person, other than contractual duties. These are different from crimes, which are defined as duty breaches against society. Many different acts can be classified as a tort or a crime, but crimes are usually prosecuted by the State, whereas torts are most often handled as a part of a lawsuit when the person has been injured.

19. C
An advance directive is a legal document filed in advance by a patient which details their wishes in the event that they are incapacitated.

Advance health care directives, which are often refused to as living wills, advance directives, advance decisions, or personal directives, are special directions given by an individual in regard to actions that are to be taken should they become unable to make decisions on their own, due to illness or incapacity, and authorizes a person to make decisions for them, with their best interests in mind. Living wills are one form of an advance directive and can leave instructions for medical treatments. Other forms authorize a very specific power of health care proxy or attorney, giving them the ability to make decisions should they become incapacitated. In some cases, both forms may be used and it is often encouraged to make sure that the patient receives the most comprehensive guidance possible when it comes to their health care. An example of this kind of combination in the United States is the Five Wishes advance directive.

20. D
The following are true about living wills:

- They are documents in which the patient chooses a

surrogate who can make healthcare decisions in the event that they are incapacitated.
- They demand that no extraordinary measures such as CPR, are used in an effort to revive the patient.

21. D
Two types of advance directives are a living will and a durable power of attorney.

Advance health care directives, sometimes referred to as a personal directive, living will, advance directive, or advance decision, are special instructions that individuals give to clarify instructions for actions to be taken should they become unable to make them. This can be due to illness, incapacitation, or other situations, and the directive will authorize another person to make decisions in their place. Living wills are a common form of advance directives and leave instructions for their treatment. Another form appoints a person to have power of attorney or health care proxy, which allows them to make the decisions pertaining to health care treatment if the patient becomes incapacitated. Many patients choose to use a combination of both forms, and this is often encouraged in order to receive the most comprehensive guidance to provide the best care. A commonly used combination in the United States is in the form of the Five Wishes advance directive.

22. A
In addition to state laws, the Uniform Anatomical Gift Act is the law that governs the donation of organs and tissues.

Organ donations, when they are to be used in transplants or as anatomical gifts of a patient's cadaver for research and dissection, are regulated by the Uniform Anatomical Gift Act. This law states that a surviving spouse, or a list of specific relatives if there is not a living spouse, can make a gift of organs without a document stating intent. This act also works to limit any liability for health care providers who are acting on good faith representations that their now deceased patient intended to make an anatomical gift if the situation should arise. This will also ban the transportation and selling of human organs in attempts to make profits from their therapy or transplants.

23. B
While negligence is a mistake or a failure to be careful, malpractice includes wrongful conduct by a professional or a failure to meet standards of care that results in harm to another person.

24. D
All of these conditions prevent organ or tissue donation:

>Advanced age and metastatic cancer
>A history of hepatitis, HIV or AIDS
>Sepsis

25. C
In whole brain death, the brain no longer functions organically and the patient is kept alive by artificial means. When a patient's cerebrum is dead and they are unconscious, cannot think or reason, but May still be breathing, they have experienced higher brain death.

Section IV – Communication and Patient Education

1. A
When communicating with another person, gestures emphasize an important point, posture can indicate either great interest or boredom, and touch can express encouragement or empathy.

2. D
A person who is crossing their arms across their chest may indicate the desire to place an unconscious barrier between themselves and others.

3. D
None of these statements are false.
Consistent eye contact can indicate a positive reaction to a speaker.

Consistent eye contact can indicate a lack of trust in the

speaker.

The use of eye contact may be dependent on the culture of the listener.

4. C
The idea of mirroring body language to put people at ease is commonly used in interviews. Mirroring the body language shows that they are understood.

5. C
The study of body language is called kinetic interpretation is false.

6. D
Nonverbal communication can signal a lack of interest or an unfriendly attitude, and can make therapeutic communication difficult to achieve.

7. B
If a patient asks a question and you do not know the answer, the best answer is always the most helpful. I.e. that you will assist them in finding the answer.

8. A
Facilitation is an important communication technique in which phrases such as "go on," please continue," and "tell me more" are used to encourage the patient.

9. B
Reflection involves repeating something the patient just said to gain more specific information and to show that you are paying attention.

10. A
The two goals of the technique of summarization are to ensure that the information that you've collected is accurate and complete and to signal the end of the interview.

11. B
Paraphrasing is restating something that a patient has said, usually in fewer words and with emphasis on the main points of their statement.

12. A
When paraphrasing is used in active listening, it demonstrates that you understand the patient's experience and allows them to evaluate their feeling by hearing them expressed by someone else.

13. A
The steps to attentive listening include, maintaining eye contact and facing the person squarely.

14. B
Facial expression, posture and tone of voice are elements of nonverbal communication.

15. D
Nonverbal communications can emphasize or contradict verbal messages is the only statement that is true.

16. C
Open-ended questions are used to obtain the most complete information available.

17. A
The statement, an interviewer should never ask close-ended questions is false. Closed-ended questions are appropriate in situations where a short answer, without elaboration is required.

18. C
Nodding provides encourages the patient to continue talking without indicating agreement or disagreement.

19. A
Using phrases that address a person's feelings, such as "You must be worried about your headaches," demonstrates empathy.

20. D
Role-playing can be an effective way to communicate with children.

Part II – Administrative Medical Assisting

Section I – Insurance

1. A
Health Maintenance Organizations, or HMOs, are organizations that are created with the intention of managing insurance contracts by working as a middle man between the insurance provider and the health care professionals, whether they be doctors, hospitals, or other professionals. Employers who have 25 employees or more are required, if they also offer traditional options for healthcare, to offer an HMO option that has been federally certified under the Health Maintenance Organization Act of 1973. This is different from traditional indemnity insurance in that it only protects care that is provided by professionals, such as doctors, who have an agreement to treat patients in a way that meets the HMO guidelines in exchange for a stream of steady patients.

2. A
In the United States, a PPO, or preferred provider organization, is an organization of hospitals, doctors, and other professional providers who have reached an agreement with third-party groups, such as insurers, to provide reduced rate care to the third-party's clients.

This is a subscription-based arrangement between the preferred provider and the insurance group. This kind of membership provides substantial savings that is well below the rates that are normally charged by the health care organization. In return, Preferred Provider Organizations also earn revenue by charging the insurer for access to their network of healthcare providers. These rates are negotiated with providers to arrange schedules of fees as well as manage any dispute that takes place between the provider and insurer.

3. B
The health care program used in the United States Department of Defence Military Health System is known as TRI-

CARE, although it was previously referred to as CHAMPUS, or the Civilian Health and Medical Program of the Uniformed Services. This service provides military retirees, personnel, their dependents, and members of the Military Reserve with civilian healthcare benefits.

4. D
The United States Government administers a social insurance program known as Medicare, which works to provide citizens 65 years of age and over with health insurance coverage. It also provides that coverage to citizens who are below the age of 65, but are disabled physically, have a congenital physical disability, or who meet a special set of criteria.

5. B
The Medicare reimbursement formula used by physicians is measured in Relative Value Units, or RVUs. These units are components of the resource-based relative value scale, or RBRVS.

6. B
An insured person's child is a dependent.

7. C
Point of service is where the service is delivered. There is also a Point Of Service insurance plan where members of a POS plan do not make a choice about which system to use until the point at which they require the service.

8. B
Pre-certification, also knows as pre-authorization. Most insurance companies require Pre-certification 24 hours before a patient is admitted or undergoes certain procedures.

9. B
Major Medical, previously known as catastrophic coverage, is a type of insurance that covers large medical charges for catastrophic and/or long illness or conditions.

10. A
Part A covers inpatient hospital stays (at least overnight), including semiprivate room, food, and tests.

Part A is responsible for coverage, when brief stays at skilled nursing facilities are required, when a specific set of criteria are met:

> 1) Any hospital stay that precedes it must last for three days or more, without including the date of discharge
> 2) The patient's stay in the nursing home must be the result of an ailment that was diagnosed either during the hospital stay, or was the reason for the stay in the hospital
> 3) The nursing home stay will be covered if the patient does not receive rehabilitation care, but does have an ailment that requires care and supervision from professionals
> 4) The nursing home must be capable of providing professional, skilled care. Part A will not cover care that is from non-skilled, custodial, or long-term care that includes activities of daily living, or ADL, such as cooking, cleaning, personal, hygiene, etc.

11. B

Part B is medical insurance for some services and products not covered by Part A, generally on an outpatient basis. Part B is optional and the beneficiary may defer if they or their spouse is still working. There is a lifetime penalty (10% per year) imposed for not enrolling in Part B unless actively working. Part B coverage begins once a patient meets his or her deductible, then typically Medicare covers 80% of approved services, while patient pays the remaining 20%.

Part B Medicare coverage pays for a variety of medical needs, such as x-rays, laboratory tests, diagnostic tests, nursing services, vaccinations, renal dialysis, ambulance transportation, outpatient hospital procedures, chemotherapy, hormonal treatments, drugs for organ transplant recipients, or other procedures that are administered inside of the patient's doctor's office. Part B also covers any medication that is administered during an office visit by the physician. Durable Medical Equipment, or DME, is also covered as part of Medicare Part B. This could be canes, walkers, mobility scooters, or wheelchairs for patients who have impairments in their mobility. It also covers prosthetic devices such as breast prosthesis after a mastectomy or artificial limbs. Finally, it can also cover a single pair of eyeglasses after a cataract surgery as well as oxygen for the home to assist with medical conditions.

12. A
TRICARE, which was previously called the Civilian Health and Medical Program of the Uniformed Services, or CHAMPUS, has been the primary care provider for the United States Military. TRICARE is responsible for providing civilian health benefits to a number of military personnel, retirees, and their dependents, as well as military Reserve members.

13. B
Workers compensation does not cover spouses. This form of medical benefits, known as Worker's Compensation, provides wage replacement, as well as the medical benefits, to any employee that has been injured during a workday and is offered as part of an agreement that the employee will not sue the employer as a tort of negligence. This bargain of compensation is an exchange between limited coverage, assured, and lack of recourse outside the system of worker compensation.

14. B
Resource-based relative value scale (RBRCS) is a schema used to determine how much money medical providers should be paid. The RBVRS is partially used by Medicare, but it is also used by almost all the HMOs, or Health Maintenance Organizations.

A physician's procedures, or a procedure by other medical providers, are assigned a value by the RBVRS and that value is adjusted by region, to fit the value of Manhattan physicians compared to El Paso physicians, for example. The assigned value can then be applied to a fixed conversion factor, which is used to determine a payment amount and changes annually.
RBVRS assigns these prices and values based on these three factors: physician procedures (52%), practice expenses (44%), and expenses for malpractice (4%).

Section II – Coding and Claims

15. C
Level III codes, also called local codes, were developed by state Medicaid agencies, Medicare contractors, and private insurers for use in specific programs and jurisdictions, for new procedures. An example might be a procedure that is covered in one State but not in another. [5]

16. C
Level III codes, also called local codes, were developed by state Medicaid agencies, Medicare contractors, and private insurers for use in specific programs and jurisdictions, for new procedures. An example might be a procedure that is covered in one State but not in another. [6]

17. B
Level II codes are alphanumeric and primarily include non-physician services such as ambulance services and prosthetic devices, and represent items and supplies and non-physician services not covered by CPT-4 codes (Level I). [6]

18. B
Level II codes are alphanumeric and primarily include non-physician services such as ambulance services and prosthetic devices, and represent items and supplies and non-physician services not covered by CPT-4 codes (Level I). [6]

19. C
Level III codes, also called local codes, were developed by state Medicaid agencies, Medicare contractors, and private insurers for use in specific programs and jurisdictions, for new procedures. An example might be a procedure that is covered in one State but not in another. [6]

20. A
All Level 1 have 5 numbers, with number ranges reserved for each of six sections, for each clinical area. [7]

21. B
Level II codes begin with a letter from A to V, followed by four numbers.

The letters at the beginning of HCPCS Level II codes have the following meaning:

- A-codes (example: A0021): Transportation, Medical & Surgical Supplies, Miscellaneous & Experimental
- B-codes (example: B4034): Enteral and Parenteral Therapy
- C-codes (example: C1300): Temporary Hospital Outpatient Prospective Payment System
- D-codes: Dental Procedures
- E-codes (example: E0100): Durable Medical Equipment
- G-codes (example: G0008): Temporary Procedures & Professional Services
- H-codes (example: H0001): Rehabilitative Services
- J-codes (example: J0120): Drugs Administered Other Than Oral Method, Chemotherapy Drugs
- K-codes (example: K0001): Temporary Codes for Durable Medical Equipment Regional Carriers
- L-codes (example: L0112): Orthotic/Prosthetic Procedures
- M-codes (example: M0064): Medical Services
- P-codes (example: P2028): Pathology and Laboratory
- Q-codes (example: Q0035): Temporary Codes
- R-codes (example: R0070): Diagnostic Radiology Services
- S-codes (example: S0012): Private Payer Codes
- T-codes (example: T1000): State Medicaid Agency Codes
- V-codes (example: V2020): Vision/Hearing Services

22. D
L-codes (example: L0112) are for Orthotic/Prosthetic Procedures

23. C
E-codes (example: E0100): Durable Medical Equipment

24. C
Level III codes, also called local codes, were developed by

state Medicaid agencies, Medicare contractors, and private insurers for use in specific programs and jurisdictions, for new procedures. An example might be a procedure that is covered in one State but not in another.

HCPCS Level III always begin with a letter from W to Z, followed by four numbers.

Section III – Finance and Bookkeeping

25. A
The Day Sheet is a daily record of services performed, charges and payments received.

26. C
The Day Sheet is an accounts receivable document.

27. B
The petty cash account is for small purchases.

28. B
The amounts of money that a company or person owes suppliers is kept in an account ledger known as Accounts Payable. This is also sometimes known as trade payables and are amounts that have not yet been paid. The office will receive an invoice, after which it is placed in the Accounts Payable until it has been paid, after which it is removed. This make it a form of credit that is offered to customers that can allow them to receive a service or product before they have actually paid for it.

29. C
A bill of lading (BL - sometimes referred to as BOL or B/L) is a document issued by a carrier to a shipper, acknowledging that specified goods have been received on board as cargo for conveyance to a named place for delivery to the consignee. The term derives from the verb "to lade" which means to load a cargo onto a ship or other form of transportation.

30. A
Accounts Receivable is money owed to a business by its cli-

ents (customers or patients) and shown on its Balance Sheet as an asset.

31. A
Superbill is itemized form utilized by healthcare providers for reflecting rendered services.

32. A
Debit and credit are the two aspects of every financial transaction. Their use and implication is the fundamental concept in the double-entry bookkeeping system, in which every debit transaction must have a corresponding credit transaction(s) and vice versa.

Debits and credits are a system of notation used in bookkeeping to determine how to record any financial transaction. In financial accounting or bookkeeping, "Dr" (Debit) means left side of a ledger account and "Cr" (Credit) is the right side of a ledger account.

33. D
Net income is the residual income of a firm after adding total revenue and gains and subtracting all expenses and losses for the reporting period.

34. B
A Bank reconciliation is a process that explains the difference between the bank balance shown in an organization's bank statement, as supplied by the bank, and the corresponding amount shown in the organization's own accounting records at a particular point in time.
Such differences may occur, for example, because

- a cheque issued by the organization has not been presented to the bank,

- a banking transaction, such as a credit received, or a charge made by the bank, has not yet been recorded in the organization's books

- either the bank or the organization itself has made an error

Part III – Clinical Medical Assisting

Section I – Asepsis

1. B
There are two types of asepsis: medical and surgical asepsis. Medical or clean asepsis reduces the number of organisms and prevents their spread. Surgical or sterile asepsis is practised by surgical technologists and nurses in operating theatres and treatment areas includes procedures to eliminate microorganisms from an area and, in an operating room, while all members of the surgical team should demonstrate good aseptic technique, it is the role of the scrub nurse or surgical technologist to set up and maintain the sterile field.

2. A
Medical Asepsis allows lotion to be applied.

3. A
Medical Asepsis requires hands to be held downwards while rinsing, while surgical asepsis requires that you hold your hands up while rinsing.

4. D
Sneezing is a means of exit for a disease to spread, not a means of transmission.

5. B
Asepsis is the state of being free from disease-causing contaminants (such as bacteria, viruses, fungi, and parasites) or, preventing contact with microorganisms.

6. C
The water temperature must be at least 2120 F and the steam temperature must be at least 2500 F for between 20 and 40 minutes.

7. B
Turning off the tap with a paper towel prevents contamination from the tap.

Section II – Vital Signs and Physical Modalities

8. C
Psychological state is not a vital sign.

9. A
98.6 F or 37 C is a normal oral temperature.

10. B
98.6 F or 37 C is a normal aural temperature.

11. B
Cryotherapy is the local or general use of low temperatures in medical therapy or the removal of heat from a body part.

12. C
Heat therapy, also called thermotherapy, is the application of heat to the body for pain relief and health. It can take the form of a hot cloth, hot water, ultrasound, heating pad, hydrocollator packs, whirlpool baths, cordless FIR heat therapy wrap, and many others.

13. C
Physical medicine and rehabilitation (PM&R), physiatry or rehabilitation medicine, is a branch of medicine that aims to enhance and restore functional ability and quality of life to those with physical impairments or disabilities.

14. A
Cryotherapy is the local or general use of low temperatures in medical therapy or the removal of heat from a body part.

15. B
Isometric exercise or isometrics are a type of strength training in which the joint angle and muscle length do not change.

16. B
Resistance exercises refer to any exercises that uses a resistance to the force of muscular contraction (also called strength training). Usually elastic or hydraulic tension provides the resistance.

17. C
In biomedical and weight lifting communities, range of motion refers to the distance and direction a joint can move between the flexed position and the extended position.

18. A
Passive exercise is movement of the body, usually of the limbs, without effort by the patient.

Section III –Clinical Pharmacology

19. A
Schedule IV

> (A) The drug or other substance has a low potential for abuse relative to the drugs or other substances in schedule III.
>
> (B) The drug or other substance has a currently accepted medical use in treatment in the United States.
>
> (C) Abuse of the drug or other substance may lead to limited physical dependence or psychological dependence relative to the drugs or other substances in schedule III.

Schedule V

> (A) The drug or other substance has a low potential for abuse relative to the drugs or other substances in schedule IV.
>
> (B) The drug or other substance has a currently accepted medical use in treatment in the United States.
>
> (C) Abuse of the drug or other substance may lead to limited physical dependence or psychological dependence relative to the drugs or other substances in schedule IV. [3]

20. A

Schedule II

(A) The drug or other substances have a high potential for abuse

(B) The drug or other substances have currently accepted medical use in treatment in the United States, or currently accepted medical use with severe restrictions

(C) Abuse of the drug or other substances may lead to severe psychological or physical dependence.

Schedule III

(A) The drug or other substance has a potential for abuse less than the drugs or other substances in schedules I and II.

(B) The drug or other substance has a currently accepted medical use in treatment in the United States.

(C) Abuse of the drug or other substance may lead to moderate or low physical dependence or high psychological dependence. [8]

21. C
Cocaine is a Schedule II drug. In general, the following are Schedule II

- Opiates
- Stimulants
- Depressants
- Cannabinoids

22. B
The drug combination diphenoxylate/atropine (trade name Lomotil) is a popular oral anti-diarrheal in the United States, manufactured by Pfizer.

23. B
An antiemetic is a drug that is effective against vomiting and nausea. Antiemetics are typically used to treat motion sickness and the side effects of opioid analgesics, general anaes-

thetics, and chemotherapy directed against cancer.

Section IV – Minor Surgery

24. A
A hemostat (also called a hemostatic clamp, arterial forceps, or pean after Jules-Émile Péan), is a vital surgical tool used in almost any surgical procedure, usually to control bleeding.

25. B
A tenaculum is a surgical instrument, usually classified as a type of forceps. It consists of a slender sharp-pointed hook attached to a handle and is used mainly in surgery for seizing and holding parts, such as blood vessels.

Uses include:

- Steadying the cervix and uterus during insertion of an intrauterine device.
- Seizing and holding as arteries in various surgical procedures.

26. B
Towel Clip

27. A
Ring Forceps

28. B
For surgical asepsis, rinse hands in an upwards position.

29. A
Always show the physician the label first.

Section V – Lab and ECG

30. A
Normal bleeding time values fall between 2 – 9 minutes depending on the method used.

31. C
The adult normal range for cholesterol (total) is 98 - 110 mEq/L.

32. A
The adult normal range reading for glucose is 80-110 mg/dL.

33. C
The normal result for a glucose reagent strip urinalysis is negative.

34. A
The normal result for a pH reagent strip urinalysis is 4.5 – 8.

35. D
The normal range for hemoglobin (Hb) is 11.7 - 16.0 g/dL.

36. B
Blood accounts for 8% of the human body weight. The average adult has a blood volume of roughly 5 liters (1.3 gal), composed of plasma and several kinds of cells.

37. A
Red blood cells are located at the bottom of a specimen tube.

38. A
Blood for glucose and alcohol testing is collected in a grey top collection tube.

39. A
The second, "atrial systole," is when the atrium contracts, the AV valves open, and blood flows from atrium to the ventricle.

40. B
The fourth, "ventricular ejection," is when the ventricles are empty and contracting, and the semilunar valves are open.

41. B
The first phase, "early diastole," is when the semilunar valves close, the atrioventricular (AV) valves open, and the whole heart is relaxed.

42. B
Complete diagram of cycles:

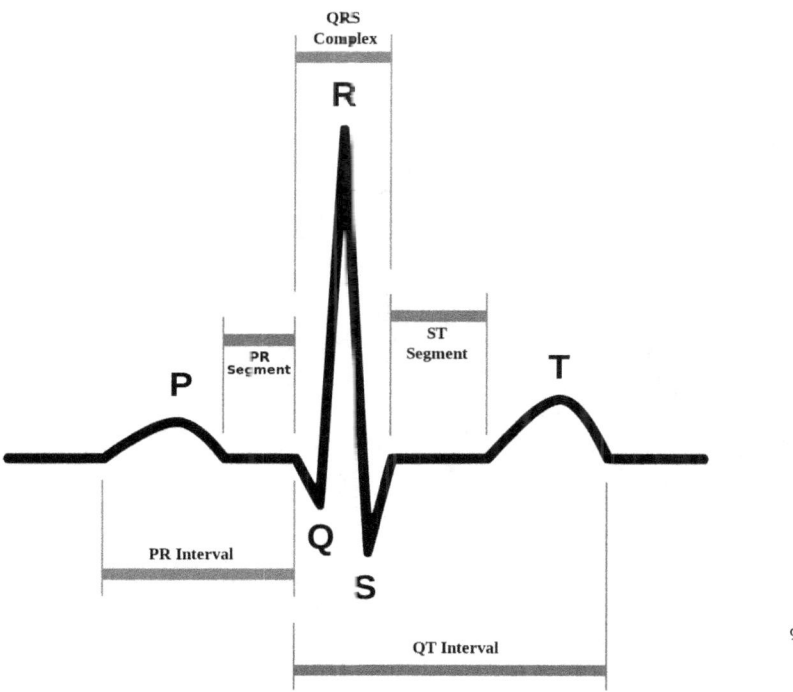

43. A
A midclavicular line (or midclavicular plane) is a vertical line crossing through the left or right clavicle.

44. A
ECG Waves and Intervals

45. A
Axillary lines

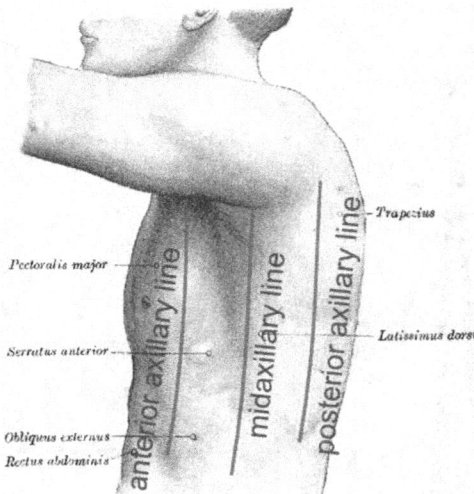

Practice Test 2

The questions below are not the same as you will find on the RMA - that would be too easy! And nobody knows what the questions will be and they change all the time. Below are general questions that cover the same subject areas as the RMA. So, while the format and exact wording of the questions may differ slightly, and change from year to year, if you can answer the questions below, you will have no problem with the RMA.

For the best results, take these Practice Test Questions as if it were the real exam. Set aside time when you will not be disturbed, and a location that is quiet and free of distractions. Read the instructions carefully, read each question carefully, and answer to the best of your ability.

Use the bubble answer sheets provided. When you have completed the Practice Questions, check your answer against the Answer Key and read the explanation provided.

Do not attempt more than one set of practice test questions in one day. After completing the first practice test, wait two or three days before attempting the second set of questions.

Part I – General Medical Assisting Knowledge

Section I – Anatomy and Physiology

1. Ⓐ Ⓑ Ⓒ Ⓓ
2. Ⓐ Ⓑ Ⓒ Ⓓ
3. Ⓐ Ⓑ Ⓒ Ⓓ
4. Ⓐ Ⓑ Ⓒ Ⓓ
5. Ⓐ Ⓑ Ⓒ Ⓓ
6. Ⓐ Ⓑ Ⓒ Ⓓ
7. Ⓐ Ⓑ Ⓒ Ⓓ
8. Ⓐ Ⓑ Ⓒ Ⓓ
9. Ⓐ Ⓑ Ⓒ Ⓓ
10. Ⓐ Ⓑ Ⓒ Ⓓ
11. Ⓐ Ⓑ Ⓒ Ⓓ
12. Ⓐ Ⓑ Ⓒ Ⓓ
13. Ⓐ Ⓑ Ⓒ Ⓓ
14. Ⓐ Ⓑ Ⓒ Ⓓ
15. Ⓐ Ⓑ Ⓒ Ⓓ
16. Ⓐ Ⓑ Ⓒ Ⓓ
17. Ⓐ Ⓑ Ⓒ Ⓓ
18. Ⓐ Ⓑ Ⓒ Ⓓ
19. Ⓐ Ⓑ Ⓒ Ⓓ
20. Ⓐ Ⓑ Ⓒ Ⓓ
21. Ⓐ Ⓑ Ⓒ Ⓓ
22. Ⓐ Ⓑ Ⓒ Ⓓ
23. Ⓐ Ⓑ Ⓒ Ⓓ
24. Ⓐ Ⓑ Ⓒ Ⓓ
25. Ⓐ Ⓑ Ⓒ Ⓓ
26. Ⓐ Ⓑ Ⓒ Ⓓ
27. Ⓐ Ⓑ Ⓒ Ⓓ
28. Ⓐ Ⓑ Ⓒ Ⓓ
29. Ⓐ Ⓑ Ⓒ Ⓓ
30. Ⓐ Ⓑ Ⓒ Ⓓ
31. Ⓐ Ⓑ Ⓒ Ⓓ
32. Ⓐ Ⓑ Ⓒ Ⓓ
33. Ⓐ Ⓑ Ⓒ Ⓓ
34. Ⓐ Ⓑ Ⓒ Ⓓ
35. Ⓐ Ⓑ Ⓒ Ⓓ
36. Ⓐ Ⓑ Ⓒ Ⓓ
37. Ⓐ Ⓑ Ⓒ Ⓓ
38. Ⓐ Ⓑ Ⓒ Ⓓ
39. Ⓐ Ⓑ Ⓒ Ⓓ
40. Ⓐ Ⓑ Ⓒ Ⓓ
41. Ⓐ Ⓑ Ⓒ Ⓓ
42. Ⓐ Ⓑ Ⓒ Ⓓ
43. Ⓐ Ⓑ Ⓒ Ⓓ
44. Ⓐ Ⓑ Ⓒ Ⓓ
45. Ⓐ Ⓑ Ⓒ Ⓓ
46. Ⓐ Ⓑ Ⓒ Ⓓ
47. Ⓐ Ⓑ Ⓒ Ⓓ
48. Ⓐ Ⓑ Ⓒ Ⓓ
49. Ⓐ Ⓑ Ⓒ Ⓓ
50. Ⓐ Ⓑ Ⓒ Ⓓ

Section II – Medical Terminology

1. Ⓐ Ⓑ Ⓒ Ⓓ   11. Ⓐ Ⓑ Ⓒ Ⓓ   21. Ⓐ Ⓑ Ⓒ Ⓓ
2. Ⓐ Ⓑ Ⓒ Ⓓ   12. Ⓐ Ⓑ Ⓒ Ⓓ   22. Ⓐ Ⓑ Ⓒ Ⓓ
3. Ⓐ Ⓑ Ⓒ Ⓓ   13. Ⓐ Ⓑ Ⓒ Ⓓ   23. Ⓐ Ⓑ Ⓒ Ⓓ
4. Ⓐ Ⓑ Ⓒ Ⓓ   14. Ⓐ Ⓑ Ⓒ Ⓓ   24. Ⓐ Ⓑ Ⓒ Ⓓ
5. Ⓐ Ⓑ Ⓒ Ⓓ   15. Ⓐ Ⓑ Ⓒ Ⓓ
6. Ⓐ Ⓑ Ⓒ Ⓓ   16. Ⓐ Ⓑ Ⓒ Ⓓ
7. Ⓐ Ⓑ Ⓒ Ⓓ   17. Ⓐ Ⓑ Ⓒ Ⓓ
8. Ⓐ Ⓑ Ⓒ Ⓓ   18. Ⓐ Ⓑ Ⓒ Ⓓ
9. Ⓐ Ⓑ Ⓒ Ⓓ   19. Ⓐ Ⓑ Ⓒ Ⓓ
10. Ⓐ Ⓑ Ⓒ Ⓓ   20. Ⓐ Ⓑ Ⓒ Ⓓ

Section III – Medical Law and Ethics

1. Ⓐ Ⓑ Ⓒ Ⓓ
2. Ⓐ Ⓑ Ⓒ Ⓓ
3. Ⓐ Ⓑ Ⓒ Ⓓ
4. Ⓐ Ⓑ Ⓒ Ⓓ
5. Ⓐ Ⓑ Ⓒ Ⓓ
6. Ⓐ Ⓑ Ⓒ Ⓓ
7. Ⓐ Ⓑ Ⓒ Ⓓ
8. Ⓐ Ⓑ Ⓒ Ⓓ
9. Ⓐ Ⓑ Ⓒ Ⓓ
10. Ⓐ Ⓑ Ⓒ Ⓓ
11. Ⓐ Ⓑ Ⓒ Ⓓ
12. Ⓐ Ⓑ Ⓒ Ⓓ
13. Ⓐ Ⓑ Ⓒ Ⓓ
14. Ⓐ Ⓑ Ⓒ Ⓓ
15. Ⓐ Ⓑ Ⓒ Ⓓ
16. Ⓐ Ⓑ Ⓒ Ⓓ
17. Ⓐ Ⓑ Ⓒ Ⓓ
18. Ⓐ Ⓑ Ⓒ Ⓓ
19. Ⓐ Ⓑ Ⓒ Ⓓ
20. Ⓐ Ⓑ Ⓒ Ⓓ

Section IV – Communication and Patient Education

1. Ⓐ Ⓑ Ⓒ Ⓓ　11. Ⓐ Ⓑ Ⓒ Ⓓ　21. Ⓐ Ⓑ Ⓒ Ⓓ
2. Ⓐ Ⓑ Ⓒ Ⓓ　12. Ⓐ Ⓑ Ⓒ Ⓓ　22. Ⓐ Ⓑ Ⓒ Ⓓ
3. Ⓐ Ⓑ Ⓒ Ⓓ　13. Ⓐ Ⓑ Ⓒ Ⓓ　23. Ⓐ Ⓑ Ⓒ Ⓓ
4. Ⓐ Ⓑ Ⓒ Ⓓ　14. Ⓐ Ⓑ Ⓒ Ⓓ　24. Ⓐ Ⓑ Ⓒ Ⓓ
5. Ⓐ Ⓑ Ⓒ Ⓓ　15. Ⓐ Ⓑ Ⓒ Ⓓ　25. Ⓐ Ⓑ Ⓒ Ⓓ
6. Ⓐ Ⓑ Ⓒ Ⓓ　16. Ⓐ Ⓑ Ⓒ Ⓓ
7. Ⓐ Ⓑ Ⓒ Ⓓ　17. Ⓐ Ⓑ Ⓒ Ⓓ
8. Ⓐ Ⓑ Ⓒ Ⓓ　18. Ⓐ Ⓑ Ⓒ Ⓓ
9. Ⓐ Ⓑ Ⓒ Ⓓ　19. Ⓐ Ⓑ Ⓒ Ⓓ
10. Ⓐ Ⓑ Ⓒ Ⓓ　20. Ⓐ Ⓑ Ⓒ Ⓓ

Part II – Administrative Medical Assisting

1. (A) (B) (C) (D)   18. (A) (B) (C) (D)
2. (A) (B) (C) (D)   19. (A) (B) (C) (D)
3. (A) (B) (C) (D)   20. (A) (B) (C) (D)
4. (A) (B) (C) (D)   21. (A) (B) (C) (D)
5. (A) (B) (C) (D)   22. (A) (B) (C) (D)
6. (A) (B) (C) (D)   23. (A) (B) (C) (D)
7. (A) (B) (C) (D)   24. (A) (B) (C) (D)
8. (A) (B) (C) (D)   25. (A) (B) (C) (D)
9. (A) (B) (C) (D)   26. (A) (B) (C) (D)
10. (A) (B) (C) (D)   27. (A) (B) (C) (D)
11. (A) (B) (C) (D)   28. (A) (B) (C) (D)
12. (A) (B) (C) (D)   29. (A) (B) (C) (D)
13. (A) (B) (C) (D)   30. (A) (B) (C) (D)
14. (A) (B) (C) (D)   31. (A) (B) (C) (D)
15. (A) (B) (C) (D)   32. (A) (B) (C) (D)
16. (A) (B) (C) (D)   33. (A) (B) (C) (D)
17. (A) (B) (C) (D)   34. (A) (B) (C) (D)

Part III – Clinical Medical Assisting

1. A B C D
2. A B C D
3. A B C D
4. A B C D
5. A B C D
6. A B C D
7. A B C D
8. A B C D
9. A B C D
10. A B C D
11. A B C D
12. A B C D
13. A B C D
14. A B C D
15. A B C D
16. A B C D
17. A B C D
18. A B C D
19. A B C D
20. A B C D
21. A B C D
22. A B C D
23. A B C D
24. A B C D
25. A B C D
26. A B C D
27. A B C D
28. A B C D
29. A B C D
30. A B C D
31. A B C D
32. A B C D
33. A B C D
34. A B C D
35. A B C D
36. A B C D
37. A B C D
38. A B C D
39. A B C D
40. A B C D
41. A B C D
42. A B C D
43. A B C D
44. A B C D
45. A B C D

Part 1 – General Medical Assisting Knowledge

Section I – Anatomy and Physiology

1. What is osteoporosis?

    a. A brain disorder that moves to the leg bones.

    b. A condition in which nerves become fragile.

    c. An ailment in which muscles deteriorate.

    d. An ailment in which bones become fragile because of loss of tissue.

2. Marfan syndrome is an example of an ailment that, rather than affecting the bones themselves, afflicts _____.

    a. The muscles.

    b. The nerves.

    c. The heart.

    d. The connective tissue.

3. Which system can be thought of as the blood distribution system?

    a. Digestive system.

    b. Musculoskeletal system.

    c. Endocrine system.

    d. Circulatory system

4. _____ are examples of nutrients passed along via the circulatory system.

    a. Citric acids
    b. Amino acids
    c. Proteins
    d. Nuclei

5. Other than blood, what else moves through the circulatory system?

    a. Traces of bone
    b. Sweat
    c. Lymph
    d. Mercury

6. What are the main components of the circulatory system?

    a. The heart, veins and blood vessels.
    b. The heart, brain, and ears.
    c. The nose, throat and ears.
    d. The lungs, stomach, and kidneys.

7. Which disease of the circulatory system is one of the most frequent causes of death in North America?

    a. The cold
    b. Pneumonia
    c. Arthritis
    d. Heart disease

8. One disease of the circulatory system, which is often mistakenly thought to be a heart attack, is _____.

    a. Cardiac arrest
    b. High blood pressure
    c. Angina
    d. Acid reflux

9. What is a more common name for the circulatory system disease known as hypertension?

    a. Anemia
    b. High blood pressure
    c. Angina
    d. Cardiac arrest

10. A condition in which the heart beats too fast, too slow, or with an irregular beat is called _____.

    a. Hypertension
    b. Angina
    c. Cardiac arrest
    d. Arrythmia

11. What is the respiratory system?

    a. The system that brings oxygen into the body and expels carbon dioxide from the body.
    b. The system that sends blood to and from the heart.
    c. The system that processes food that enters the body.
    d. The system that expels urine from the body.

12. Which of the following is an example of an important component of the respiratory system?

    a. The cornea
    b. The lungs
    c. The kidneys
    d. The stomach

13. The exchange of oxygen for carbon dioxide takes place in the alveolar area of _____

    a. The throat.
    b. The ears.
    c. The appendix.
    d. The lungs.

14. The part of the body that initiates inhalation is _____

    a. The lungs.
    b. The diaphragm.
    c. The larynx.
    d. The kidneys.

15. Exhalation is often accomplished by _____ .

    a. Abdominal muscles
    b. Chest muscles.
    c. The esophagus.
    d. The nasal passageway.

16. What is the primary thing oxygenated through the work of the respiratory system?

    a. The brain
    b. The limbs
    c. The heart
    d. The blood

17. An example of an important side-benefit of the respiratory system is

    a. The air allows whistling.
    b. The oxygen expelled can be recycled for other uses.
    c. The air being expelled from the mouth allows for speaking.
    d. The air expelled from the body also expels disease and germs.

18. An example of a disease of the lungs that is caused or made worse by smoking is _____.

    a. Emphysema.
    b. Strep throat.
    c. Muscular dystrophy.
    d. Leukemia.

19. The immune system is _____.

    a. The system that expels waste from the body.
    b. The system that expels carbon dioxide from the body.
    c. The system that protects the body from disease and infection.
    d. The system that circulates blood through the body.

20. How does the immune system fight off disease?

    a. By identifying and killing tumor cells and pathogens.
    b. By creating new blood cells that fight disease.
    c. By expelling infection through the blood stream.
    d. By giving you energy to resist disease infections.

21. An example of a pathogen that the immune system detects is _____.

    a. An atom.
    b. A molecule.
    c. A vitamin.
    d. A virus.

22. Detection of pathogens can be complicated because _____.

    a. They evolve so quickly.
    b. They die so quickly.
    c. They are invisible.
    d. They multiply so quickly.

23. One of the best-known disorders that attack the immune system is _____.

    a. Rabies
    b. HIV (the virus that causes AIDS)
    c. Lung cancer
    d. Muscular dystrophy

24. The process by which the immune system adapts over time to be more efficient in recognizing pathogens is known as _____.

    a. Acquired immunity
    b. AIDS
    c. Pathogens
    d. Acquired deficiency

25. _____ is an example of an early response by the immune system to infection.

    a. Inhalation
    b. Inflammation
    c. Respiration
    d. Exhalation.

26. Which cells are an important weapon in the fight against infection?

    a. Red blood cells
    b. White blood cells
    c. Barrier cells
    d. Virus cells

27. What is the primary purpose of the digestive system?

    a. To expel food and liquids from the body.
    b. To absorb oxygen from food.
    c. To help circulate blood throughout the body.
    d. To convert food into a form that can provide nourishment for the body.

28. An important element in the digestive process is the _____ that help break down the food.

    a. Digestive juices
    b. Proteins
    c. Amino acids
    d. Chromosomes

29. Where does digestion begin?

    a. In the throat.
    b. In the stomach.
    c. In the intestines.
    d. In the mouth.

30. Which of these is not an example of a function of the stomach in digestion?

    a. Storing food.
    b. Cleansing food of impurities.
    c. Mixing food with digestive juices.
    d. Transferring food into the intestines.

31. _____ are the kinds of food that stay in the stomach longest.

    a. Fats
    b. Proteins
    c. Carbohydrates
    d. Vitamins

32. One common digestive affliction that most people suffer at one time or other is _____.

    a. Stomach cancer
    b. Ulceritis
    c. Indigestion
    d. The flu

33. When a pouch in the large intestine becomes inflamed, this becomes an affliction known as _____.

    a. Diverticulosis
    b. Diverticulitis
    c. Acid Reflux
    d. Colon Cancer

34. The best way to avoid most digestive diseases is _____.

    a. Eating a healthy diet.
    b. Eating only proteins.
    c. Never eating dessert.
    d. Trying not to get angry.

35. The three functions of the urinary system are _____.

    a. Taking in oxygen, distributing oxygen, and helping the heart to relax.
    b. Cleansing the blood stream, sending blood throughout the body, and fighting disease.
    c. Improving lung function, improving stomach function and improving the heart rate.
    d. Producing, storing and eliminating urine.

36. What is mostly true of urine?

a. It's mostly comprised of healthy vitamins and nutrients.

b. It's mostly comprised of waste material after the body has taken the nutrients from food and absorbed the water it needs.

c. It's mostly useless in the body.

d. It's mostly carbohydrates.

37. _____ is the name of the waste removed from the body through urine.

a. Urea

b. Urinalysis

c. Feces

d. Fat

38. One example of the blood stream's part in the digestive system is _____.

a. Preventing infection.

b. Carrying urea to the kidneys.

c. Expelling the urea from the body.

d. The blood stream has no part in the digestive system.

39. Besides the kidney, the other major organ that takes part in the body's urinary system is _____.

a. The Penis

b. The Liver

c. The Stomach

d. The Bladder

40. Which of these describes the bladder?

a. A pea-sized, circular organ.

b. A balloon shaped, muscular organ.

c. A squarish organ about the size of the small intestine.

d. A triangular organ the same size as the heart.

41. An example of one of the many serious urinary disorders is _____.

a. Liver failure

b. Stomach ulcer

c. Kidney failure

d. Lung cancer

42. The involuntary passage of urine defines the urinary-system disorder known as _____.

a. Incontinence

b. Impotence

c. Bladder cancer

d. Stomach ulcer

43. The lymphatic system is the system which _____.

a. Carries a clear liquid ("lymph") toward the heart.

b. Carries a clear liquid ("lymph") out through the bowels.

c. Heals the lymph nodes.

d. Cleanses the blood stream of bacteria.

44. Which of these is true of lymphoid tissue?

a. It exists only in the lymph nodes.

b. It exists in many organs, although it's predominantly in the lymph nodes.

c. Humans have evolved beyond having lymphoid tissue in their bodies.

d. Lymphoid tissue is always cancerous.

45. An example of an organ that plays a big role in the lymphatic system is _____.

a. The spine.
b. The kidney
c. The spleen.
d. The liver.

46. Among the benefits of the lymphatic system is the fact that it _____.

a. Has no known benefit.

b. Removes most cancerous material from the body.

c. Removes urine and feces from the body.

d. Absorbs and transports fats and fatty acids from the body's circulatory system.

47. Which of these defines "metastasis?"

a. Process of carrying cancer cells between various parts of the body.

b. Process of eliminating all cancer cells.

c. Process of expelling bodily waste from the body.

d. Process in which a benign tumor becomes cancerous.

48. A common affliction of the lymphatic system is _____.

    a. Disintegration of the lymph nodes.
    b. Swelling of the lymph nodes.
    c. Constipation
    d. Ear / Nose problems.

49. An example of a cause of lymph node swelling is _____.

    a. Infectious mononucleosis ("Mono")
    b. The flu
    c. Arthritis
    d. Appendicitis

50. Another, more serious, example of a cause of lymph node swelling is _____.

    a. Tuberculosis
    b. Muscular dystrophy
    c. Multiple sclerosis
    d. Cancer

Section II – Medical Terminology

1. Bodily organs can sometimes adhere to the _____, a two-layered membrane lining the abdominal cavity and covering abdominal organs; when this occurs, the problem is corrected through surgical release of _____ adhesions.

   a. Bodily organs can sometimes adhere to the peritoneum, a two-layered membrane lining the abdominal cavity and covering abdominal organs; when this occurs, it the problem is corrected through surgical release of peritoneal adhesions.

   b. Bodily organs can sometimes adhere to the adipose tissue, a two-layered membrane lining the abdominal cavity and covering abdominal organs; when this occurs, the problem is corrected through surgical release of adipose adhesions.

   c. Bodily organs can sometimes adhere to the perumbilicus, a two-layered membrane lining the abdominal cavity and covering abdominal organs; when this occurs, the problem is corrected through surgical release of perumbilicus adhesions.

   d. Bodily organs can sometimes adhere to the perilingual, a two-layered membrane lining the abdominal cavity and covering abdominal organs; when this occurs, the problem is corrected through surgical release of perilingual adhesions.

2. A/an _____ allows a physician to obtain a small, representative sample of tissue for microscopic examination; this is usually done to establish a diagnosis.

   a. Laparoscopy
   b. Endarterectomy
   c. Biopsy
   d. CRT

3. Which surgery is indicated when part of the intestine protrudes into the groin?

   a. Inguinal hernia repair
   b. Colectomy
   c. Adhesion repair
   d. Prostatectomy

4. _____ are distended veins in the lower rectum or anus; a/an _____ is performed to relieve this condition.

   a. Mastoids are distended veins in the lower rectum or anus; a mastectomy is performed to relieve this condition.
   b. Flavonoids are distended veins in the lower rectum or anus; a flavonoidectomy is performed to relieve this condition.
   c. Hemorrhoids are distended veins in the lower rectum or anus; a hemorrhoidectomy is performed to relieve this condition.
   d. Tumoroids are distended veins in the lower rectum or anus; a tumorectomy is performed to relieve this condition.

5. During _____, a tight band of transverse fibrous tissue is cut, releasing pressure on the median nerves and relieving symptoms.

   a. Adhesion repair surgery
   b. Open carpal tunnel surgery
   c. Carotid surgery
   d. Ligament surgery

6. A surgical procedure that unblocks the arteries located in the neck which supply blood to the brain is a/an _____.

    a. Carotid endarterectomy
    b. Arterial cleanse
    c. Peripheral endarterectomy
    d. Colectomy

7. _____ involves removal of the opaque contents of a lens of the eye via ultrasound waves, although, in some cases, the entire lens is removed and replaced with an artificial lens.

    a. Vitrectomy surgery
    b. Retinopathy surgery
    c. Laser surgery
    d. Cataract surgery

8. Which, if any, of the following statements concerning hysterectomies are false?

    a. A hysterectomy is the surgical removal of the uterus.
    b. A hysterectomy can be performed through either an abdominal incision or vaginally.
    c. Following a radical hysterectomy, a small number of patients are placed on a hormone replacement regimen.
    d. A radical hysterectomy includes the removal of the uterus, tubes, ovaries, adjacent lymph nodes and a portion of the vagina.

9. Which, if any, of the following statements about fluoroscopy are false?

   a. Fluoroscopy utilizes a continuous or pulsed bean of low-dose radiation.

   b. Fluoroscopy is a type of x-ray that can be used to evaluate the flow of blood through the arteries.

   c. Fluoroscopy produces a series of still images of the body part being examined.

   d. Images can be videotaped or sent to a monitor for viewing.

10. A/an _____ is a test employed to identify blockages in the circulatory system, diagnose stroke and determine the size and location of brain tumors and aneurysms.

   a. Angiogram

   b. Arterial fluid analysis

   c. Ultrasound imaging

   d. None of the above.

11. During a _____, a small sample of tissue is removed, usually under local anesthetic, examined microscopically for diagnosis.

   a. Amniocentesis

   b. Biopsy

   c. Cerebrospinal analysis

   d. Culture

12. What areas of dysfunction are diagnosed through the use of electromyography?

   a. Nerve and muscle dysfunction and spinal cord disease

   b. Balance disorders and hearing loss

   c. Arrhythmia and tachycardia

   d. None of the above

13. Which, if any, of the following statements about cerebrospinal fluid analysis (CSF) are false?

a. CSF are tests that measure proteins, glucose and other chemicals contained in the fluid that protects the brain and spinal cord.

b. A lumbar puncture is performed to obtain a fluid sample, a painless procedure completed without the use of anesthetic.

c. CSF analysis can be used to diagnose infections (such as meningitis) and brain or spinal cord damage, as well as to measure intracranial pressure.

d. Some cases of multiple sclerosis can be detected through CSF.

14. _____, also known as a _____, is used to detect bone and vascular anomalies, certain types of brain tumors, and blood clots in patients who have experienced a stroke or brain damage due to an injury.

a. Electroencephalography, EEG

b. Electromyography, EMG

c. Positron emission tomography, PET

d. Computed tomography, CT scan

15. Using the magnetic properties of the blood, a _____ produces real-time images of blood flow to certain areas of the brain and assesses damage due to head injury or disorders such as Alzheimer's disease.

a. Positron emission tomography

b. Ultrasound imaging

c. Electroencephalography

d. Functional MRI (fMRI)

16. Which, if any, of the following statements about positron emission tomography (PET) scans are false?

   a. Before the test, a low-level radioactive isotope is injected into the patient's bloodstream.

   b. PET scans are used to detect tumors and measure cellular metabolism.

   c. PET scans are frequently used instead of CT or MRI scans, which are significantly less accurate.

   d. Alterations in the brain as a result of damage or drug use can be determined through a PET scan.

17. The goal of _____, also called physiatry, is to enhance and restore functional ability to those with disabilities or physical impairments.

   a. Rheumatology

   b. Physical medicine and rehabilitation

   c. Orthopedic medicine

   d. Immunology

18. _____ is a branch of medicine concerned with diseases of the rectum, anus, colon and pelvic floor.

   a. Urology

   b. Nephrology

   c. Immunology

   d. Proctology

19. Which, of any, of the following statement concerning pulmonology are true?

   a. Pulmonology is also called pneumology.

   b. The focus of this specialty is the diagnosis of lung diseases, as well as the prevention of secondary diseases such as tuberculosis.

   c. Pulmonology is closely associated with critical care medicine in that it deals with patients who require mechanical ventilation.

   d. All of the above.

20. Which branch of medicine centers around the treatment of conditions affecting joints, muscles, and bones, as well as some autoimmune diseases and vasculitis?

    a. Immunology

    b. Rheumatology

    c. Angiology

    d. Rehabilitative medicine

21. _____ medicine, known in Europe as angiology, is a medical specialty centered on the study of the _____ and _____ systems and diseases associated with those systems.

    a. Vascular medicine, known in Europe as angiology, is a medical specialty centered on the study of the circulatory and lymphatic systems and diseases associated with those systems.

    b. Thoracic medicine, known in Europe as angiology, is a medical specialty centered on the study of the circulatory and lymphatic systems and diseases associated with those systems.

    c. Vascular medicine, known in Europe as angiology, is a medical specialty centered on the study of the respiratory and circulatory systems and diseases associated with those systems.

    d. Physical medicine, known in Europe as angiology, is a medical specialty centered on the study of the circulatory and lymphatic systems and diseases associated with those systems.

22. Which, if any, of the following statements about thoracic surgery are false?

   a. Thoracic surgeons treat diseases that affect the organs within the chest.

   b. Treatment most frequently involves conditions of the lungs, chest wall and diaphragm.

   c. Many times, thoracic surgery is grouped with cardiac surgery and termed cardiothoracic surgery.

   d. All of these statements are true.

23. _____ is both a medical and surgical specialty focused on the urinary tracts of both men and women and the reproductive systems of males.

   a. Nephrology
   b. Urology
   c. Andrology
   d. Endocrinology

24. _____ surgery is surgery performed on the heart and/or major blood vessels to treat complications of ischemic heart disease, correct congenital heart disease, etc.

   a. Cardiothoracic
   b. Angiologic
   c. Cardiovascular
   d. Transplant

Section III – Medical Law and Ethics

1. As a/an _____, you are required by law to report the abuse or neglect of a child, despite the fact that such a report breaches confidentiality.

    a. Third party
    b. Concerned citizen
    c. Mandated reporter
    d. Impartial witness

2. **Signs of physical child abuse include:**

    a. Flinching at sudden movements
    b. Non-attachment to parent
    c. Poor hygiene
    d. Sudden changes in weight or appetite

3. **Signs of emotional abuse include:**

    a. Non-attachment to parent
    b. Seductive behavior
    c. Poor hygiene
    d. Clothing inappropriate for the season

4. **Signs of sexual abuse include:**

    a. Problems sitting or walking
    b. Running away from home
    c. Pregnancy or STD under the age of 14
    d. All of the above

5. _____ is a pattern of not caring for a child, either physically or emotionally, that threatens the child's well-being.

   a. Sexual abuse
   b. Emotional abuse
   c. Physical abuse
   d. Child neglect

6. Fetal abuse has become an important and highly publicized issue in recent years. Which, if any, of the following are indications of fetal abuse?

   a. Poor fetal growth on abdomen measurements or ultrasound
   b. History or signs of domestic abuse
   c. History or signs of maternal alcohol or drug use
   d. All of the above

7. Which of the following statements are used by the Uniform Determination of Death Act (UDDA) to define death?

   a. The individual has sustained irreversible cessation of circulatory and respiratory functions.
   b. The individual has sustained irreversible cessation of all functions of the entire brain, including the brain stem.
   c. The person has lost their capacity for reasoning, self-awareness, communication, agency, and consciousness of the external world.
   d. Both a. and b.

8. _____ is defined as performing an act that one should not do at all or the unjust performance of such an act.

   a. Malpractice
   b. Malfeasance
   c. Misdemeanor
   d. A Lapse in judgment

9. According to the Health Information Portability and Accountability Act (HIPAA), which, if any, of these persons/organizations are allowed limited or full access to a patient's medical records?

   a. Family, even if the patient is fully competent and in charge of their affairs
   b. Close personal friends or life partners
   c. Government agencies such as Medicare, Workers Compensation and Social Security Disability Insurance
   d. None of the above

10. Under which of the following conditions, if any, can the medical information of a person at risk for HIV be released without patient permission?

    a. In an emergency situation to medical personnel or a court order has been issued
    b. For the purpose of review board approved research
    c. If the spouse has requested the information
    d. Unless patient permission has been given, medical information cannot be released under any conditions.

11. _____ refers to what society owes a person in proportion to their individual needs and responsibilities, the resources available and society's responsibilities to the common good.

    a. Ethical distribution
    b. Distributive justice
    c. Benevolent justice
    d. Egalitarian ethics

12. A system of health care in which patients agree to visit only certain doctors and hospitals, and in which the cost of treatment is monitored is called _____.

    a. Managed care
    b. Private care
    c. Medicaid and Medicare
    d. Socialized medicine

13. Which of these statements regarding the medical treatment of illegal immigrants are true?

    a. In the United States, healthcare is not rationed by citizenship.

    b. The Illegal Immigration Reform and Immigrant Responsibility Act states that illegal immigrants are forbidden from receiving healthcare through Medicaid and Medicare with the exception of pregnancy care.

    c. The use of citizenship to ration healthcare violates the principle of benevolence.

    d. None of these statements are true.

14. A _____ indicates that a patient does not want cardiopulmonary resuscitation or defibrillation at the end of life, while a _____ order indicates that the patient rejects the use of a breathing tube in cases of respiratory arrest. _____ can be _____ at any time.

    a. A living will indicates that a patient does not want cardiopulmonary resuscitation or defibrillation at the end of life, while a DNI order indicates that the patient rejects the use of a breathing tube in cases of respiratory arrest. Both can be revoked at any time.

    b. A Do Not Resuscitate (DNR) indicates that a patient does not want cardiopulmonary resuscitation or defibrillation at the end of life while a DNI order indicates that the patient rejects the use of a breathing tube in cases of respiratory arrest. Neither can be revoked at any time.

    c. A Do Not Resuscitate (DNR) indicates that a patient does not want cardiopulmonary resuscitation or defibrillation at the end of life, while a DNI order indicates that the patient rejects the use of a breathing tube in cases of respiratory arrest. Both can be revoked at any time.

    d. A DNI order indicates that a patient does not want cardiopulmonary resuscitation or defibrillation at the end of life while a Do Not Resuscitate (DNR) indicates that the patient rejects the use of a breathing tube in cases of respiratory arrest. Both can be revoked at any time.

15. _____ is a legal term meaning that the patient has the mental and legal ability to make decisions.

    a. Autonomy

    b. Fitness

    c. Competence

    d. Common sense

16. In the United States, _____ refers to legal actions that cannot result in a person being punished by imprisonment.

 a. Criminal law
 b. Civil law
 c. Cause of action
 d. Comparative negligence

17. _____ refers to an ability to interact effectively with people of different _____.

 a. Religious aptitude refers to an ability to interact effectively with people of different faiths.
 b. Cultural diversity refers to an ability to interact effectively with people of different cultures.
 c. Ethnic forbearance refers to an ability to interact effectively with people of different ethnicities.
 d. Cultural competence refers to an ability to interact effectively with people of different cultures.

18. _____ are the most common type of treatment error.

 a. Medication errors
 b. Surgical errors
 c. Improper uses of medical equipment
 d. Misinterpretations of lab results

19. Types of medication errors include:

 a. Administration errors which occur when the provider gives the wrong medicine to the patient
 b. Pharmacy fulfillment errors
 c. Transcription errors which occur when the pharmacist misreads the prescription or it is written incorrectly
 d. All of the above

Practice Test Questions Set 2

20. Which, if any, of the following statements about ethics and legality are true?

a. The law demands that patients are treated compassionately, while ethics require competent medical practice according to current standards and frequently exceed legal standards.

b. Breaches of ethics are usually not legally enforceable.

c. Ethics set rigid conduct standards that must be met while laws set flexible guidelines for conduct.

d. None of the above are true.

21. According to the tenets of the Americans with Disabilities Act, a medical professional cannot:

a. Charge excessively high fees.

b. Refuse to respond in emergency situations.

c. Terminate patient care in the middle of treatment.

d. Refuse to treat a patient with an infectious disease.

22. _____ is a federal law intended to standardize healthcare information and its use in the United States.

a. The Americans with Disabilities Act

b. The AMT Code of Ethics

c. The Health Information Portability and Accountability Act

d. The Protected Health Information Act

23. Which, if any, of the following statements about the patient rights of adolescents is true?

   a. All 50 states allow minors to be tested for STDs, including HIV, without parental permission.

   b. Informed consent forms must be written at the minor's level.

   c. Adolescents must always obtain parental permission before placing a child for adoption.

   d. In most states, minors may apply to a judge for a confidential alteration, which allows them to obtain an abortion without parental consent or notification.

24. An emancipated minor:

   a. Is a person who, although not having reached the statutory age of majority, is granted the legal status of an adult

   b. Is an adolescent who given birth to a child.

   c. Can be living with and supported by their parents.

   d. Has received approval for the action from their guardians.

25. A _____ is a person who has a duty to act primarily for another's benefit, as a trustee; this phrase also pertains the good faith and confidence involved in such a relationship.

   a. Fiduciary

   b. Guardian

   c. Advocate

   d. Sponsor

Section IV – Communication Skills and Patient Education

1. Which of the following can act as a barrier to communication?

    a. Attention

    b. Level of education

    c. Families

    d. Age

2. _____ is the zone around each person reserved for _____ and can vary according to _____.

    a. Personal space is the zone around each person reserved for conversation and can vary according to culture.

    b. Intimate space is the zone around each person reserved for conversation and can vary according to culture.

    c. Personal space is the zone around each person reserved for conversation and can vary according to age.

    d. Inner space is the zone around each person reserved for conversation and can vary according to culture.

3. When dealing with elderly patients, always _____.

    a. Use their first names to establish intimacy.

    b. Direct your questions to their caregivers.

    c. Speak loudly and distinctly.

    d. Address them as Miss, Mrs., or Mr., followed by their last name.

4. A complete medical history should include:

   a. Insurance information
   b. The chief complaint
   c. Marital history
   d. All of the above

5. When documenting a patient's chief complaint, be careful to _____.

   a. Use the appropriate medical terms.
   b. Base your notes on comments from the family.
   c. Use the patient's exact words.
   d. None of the above.

6. Physical barriers to communication include:

   a. Time
   b. Environment
   c. Illness
   d. All of the above

7. If a patient does not seem to understand a question:

   a. Repeat the question using simpler terms.
   b. Ask them if they understood the question.
   c. Skip the question and come back to it later.
   d. Base your note on their medical history.

8. The interviewer says, "I want to be sure that I understand what you've said. You've been having headaches for several weeks, but you thought they would just go away on their own." The interviewer is using the interview technique of _____.

    a. Summarizing
    b. Paraphrasing
    c. Edifying
    d. Perception checking

9. For patients who are depressed, cognitively impaired, or unable to deal with complex communication at that particular moment, using _____ that require short answers can help obtain information.

    a. Indirect questions
    b. Feedback
    c. Direct questions
    d. Paraphrasing

10. Which, if any, of the following statements about the issue of silence during an interview are false?

    a. While beneficial to the interview process, silence can sometimes be perceived as a lack of interest.
    b. Silence should always be avoided in the interview process.
    c. Silence allows the patient to think about their answer to a question.
    d. Silence can be broken by short comments that do not require a response.

11. "You've been feeling depressed, haven't you?" is an example of a/an _____.

   a. Indirect question
   b. Direct question
   c. Leading question
   d. Feedback

12. Leading questions are an ineffective means of obtaining information because:

   a. The patient may feel forced to give the answer the interviewer is looking for.
   b. The patient may not understand the question.
   c. The response is likely to be either short or unclear.
   d. Asking a leading question is illegal.

13. During the interview process, the most accurate information is provided by _____.

   a. Medical records
   b. Family members
   c. Close friends
   d. The patient

14. When interviewing a patient with a hearing loss, remember to _____.

   a. Speak slowly and look directly at the patient.
   b. Ensure that the room is brightly lit.
   c. Write down your questions and have them write their answers.
   d. Both a) and b).

15. _____ is the key means of communication between healthcare workers.

    a. Email
    b. The telephone
    c. Conversation
    d. The medical record

16. A/an _____ is used to obtain _____ information and learn about past and current health problems.

    a. An interview is used to obtain insurance information and learn about past and current health problems.
    b. A health history is used to obtain subjective information and learn about past and current health problems.
    c. A biography is used to obtain sufficient information and learn about past and current health problems.
    d. A diagnostic procedure is used to obtain subjective information and learn about past and current health problems.

17. What is the first area to be covered when obtaining a health history?

    a. Chief complaint
    b. Insurance coverage
    c. Biographical information
    d. Family history

18. Using neutral remarks such as, "I see" and "I hear what you're saying" indicate _____ to the patient.

    a. Empathy
    b. Recognition
    c. Understanding
    d. Avoidance

19. In addition to providing _____ patient information to other healthcare professionals, it is necessary that one be able to _____ what others have added to the medical record.

> a. In addition to providing objective patient information to other healthcare professionals, it is necessary that one be able to increase what others have added to the medical record.
>
> b. In addition to providing legible patient information to other healthcare professionals, it is necessary that one be able to read what others have added to the medical record.
>
> c. In addition to providing accurate patient information to other healthcare professionals, it is necessary that one be able to discuss what others have added to the medical record.
>
> d. In addition to providing accurate patient information to other healthcare professionals, it is necessary that one be able to interpret what others have added to the medical record.

20. If a patient refuses to make eye contact, you may find that they are _____.

> a. From a culture that considers direct eye contact rude.
>
> b. Very tired.
>
> c. Lying about their symptoms.
>
> d. Disinterested in the conversation.

Part II – Administrative Medical Assisting

Section I – Insurance

1. **What is the birthday rule?**

    a. Methods to determine the primary insurance carrier when both parent's policy cover dependents.

    b. A method to determine the primary insurance carrier when both parents are covered.

    c. A method to determine the primary insurance carrier eligibility

    d. A method to determine the primary insurance carrier fees

2. **What type of insurance generally covers workplace accidents?**

    a. Medicare

    b. TRICARE

    c. Workers Compensation

    d. Patient's primary insurance carrier

3. **What is an EOB?**

    a. classification of diagnoses

    b. method to determine coverage

    c. a relative value unit

    d. a summary of services covered.

4. What is a method used by insurance carriers to determine prices based on prices charge by other carriers?

    a. Usual, Customary and Reasonable
    b. Reasonable Fee determination
    c. Usual Carrier Fees
    d. None of the Above

5. What is the process of determining how much or if the primary carrier will pay for a service?

    a. Predetermination
    b. Pre-certification
    c. Fee Quote
    d. None of the Above

6. What is the UCR fee of providers in an area called?

    a. Prevailing fee
    b. Customary fee
    c. Usual fee
    d. Local fee

7. What type of insurance carrier typically allows insured persons to select their own health care provider?

    a. Indemnity
    b. HMO
    c. Blue Cross
    d. TRICARE

8. What part of Medicare allows choice of a Medicare Advantage Plan?

    a. Part A

    b. Part B

    c. Part C

    d. Medicare does not allow choice of Medicare Advantage Plan

9. What is an Assignment of Benefits?

    a. Authorization for the insurance company to send payments to the provider

    b. Authorization for the insurance company to send payments to the insured person's spouse

    c. Authorization for the insurance company to send payments to a deceased persons dependent

    d. Authorization for the provider to perform the service

10. What is RVS?

    a. The system for reimbursement

    b. The relative values listed by procedure code

    c. The component multiplied by a factor to calculate cost

    d. None of the Above

11. What is Co-payment?

    a. Portion of total cost the insured person must pay

    b. Portion of total cost paid by a spouses' insurance

    c. Portion of total cost paid by the health care provider

    d. Portion of total cost paid by the primary insurance carrier

12. What are diagnostic-related groups (DRG)?

a. Classification of diagnoses to determine hospital payment under Medicare

b. Classification of procedures to determine hospital payment under Medicare

c. Classification of diagnoses to determine hospital payment under TRICARE

d. Classification of diagnoses to determine insured payment under Medicare

13. What is Pre-certification?

a. Determining if a service is authorized.

b. Calculating the amount the carrier will pay for a service.

c. Obtaining approval for a service in advance.

d. Determining if a service is covered.

14. What is a third-party payer?

a. Whoever pays the doctor or hospital for the serviced given to the patient.

b. Whoever pays the patient for the services given by the doctor or hospital.

c. Whoever pays the primary carrier for the services provided to the patient.

d. None of the Above

Section II – Coding and Claims

15. What is the process where several CPT codes are used for a procedure that is normally covered by 1 code?

    a. Unbundling

    b. Split Billing

    c. Yo-yoing

    d. None of the Above

16. What section of the CPT contains codes from 10000 to 69999 and is the largest?

    a. Medicine

    b. Anesthesia

    c. Radiology

    d. Surgery

17. Which Diagnostic codes identify encounters other than illness or injury?

    a. ICD-9 Numerical

    b. ICD-9 E codes

    c. ICD-9 V codes

    d. ICD-9 S codes

18. Dirty Claims are:

    a. claims rejected by the insurance company due to errors or other reasons.

    b. claims rejected by the healthcare provider due to errors or other reasons.

    c. fraudulent claims

    d. criminal fraudulent claims

19. Split billing refers to:

　　a. Splitting the billing between two insurance carriers.
　　b. Billing for several visits when only one visit occurred.
　　c. Splitting the billing between two physicians.
　　d. Splitting the billing between two healthcare providers.

20. What is a CMS 1500?

　　a. A term used in ICD-9 coding.
　　b. A term used in Current Procedural Terminology coding.
　　c. The universal health care claim form.
　　d. A term used in HCPCS coding.

21. What is etiology?

　　a. A type of disease
　　b. A type of procedure
　　c. The cause of disease
　　d. None of the Above

22. The HCPCS Level II code for Chemotherapy Drugs is:

　　a. P-codes
　　b. G-codes
　　c. J-codes
　　d. L-codes

23. The HCPCS Level II code for Temporary Procedures & Professional Services is:

　　a. G-codes
　　b. L-codes
　　c. E-codes
　　d. M-codes

24. E code classification of the ICD-9 is for:

   a. external injuries

   b. emergency room treatments

   c. any emergency treatment

   d. E codes are not part of the ICD-9 coding system

Section III – Finance and Bookkeeping

25. What contains a listing of patients and amounts owing

   a. Day sheet

   b. General Ledger

   c. Pegboard system

   d. Account Receivable ledger

26. When a refund is made to a patient it is a(n)

   a. Adjustment

   b. Charge

   c. Receivable

   d. None of the Above

27. Monitoring overdue accounts is called

   a. Reconciling

   b. Auditing

   c. Aging accounts

   d. Checking

28. Accounts payable are considered a(n)

a. Asset
b. Liability
c. Neither Asset nor Liability

29. A customer check returned or bounced by the bank will be marked

a. ISF
b. NSF
c. Bounced
d. Returned

30. An endorsement is

a. A signature on the front of a check
b. A signature on the back of a check
c. An initial on a check
d. A signature on a contract

31. What is the tax withheld for Social Security and Medicare called?

a. Social Security and Health Act (SSHA)
b. Federal Insurance and Contribution Act (FICA)
c. Federal Income tax
d. Health and Security Act (HAS)

32. A purchase order

a. Is sent by the supplier to the medical office
b. Is sent by the medical office to a supplier
c. Is required by most insurance companies
d. None of the Above

33. The doctor has requested a discount for a patient. This is called

    a. Account Receivable
    b. Account Payable
    c. Adjustment
    d. None of the Above.

34. A check is not used or filled out in error. What should you do?

    a. Tear out and discard
    b. Mark Void
    c. Leave in check book
    d. None of the above

Part III – Clinical Medical Assisting

Section I – Asepsis

1. What federal agency develops and monitors standards for workplace health and safety?

    a. FDA
    b. ADA
    c. OSHA
    d. None of the Above

2. All of the following are susceptible hosts except:

    a. Patient with depressed immunity
    b. Patient with no immunity
    c. Poor nutrition
    d. Normal immunity

3. How do you know an autoclave has finished sterilizing?

    a. The timer is at zero

    b. The pressure gauge is zero

    c. Both the timer and pressure gauge are zero

    d. The autoclave is cool to touch

4. The most important standard precaution is

    a. Treat all bodily fluids as contaminated

    b. Wear gloves as much as possible

    c. Only wear gloves when you think a patient is contaminated

    d. Always label specimens immediately

5. When a patient is infected in a health care facility

    a. causative

    b. Nosocomial

    c. No special name

    d. Pathogenic

6. Influenza is caused by

    a. A fungus

    b. Bacteria

    c. A virus

    d. Protozoa

7. Which of the following is not a type of pathogen?

    a. Virus

    b. Lichen

    c. Fungus

    d. Protozoa

Section II – Vital Signs and Physical Modalities

8. What is the normal adult pulse?

    a. 70 to 120 bpm
    b. 60 to 100 bps
    c. 100 - 120 bpm
    d. 60 to 100 bpm

9. What anatomic site is used to measure circulation to the extremities?

    a. Popliteal
    b. Brachial
    c. Apical
    d. Femoral

10. What is a regular rate of respiration for an adult?

    a. 10 - 15 cycles per minute
    b. 12 to 20 cycles per minute
    c. 15 to 20 cycles per minute
    d. 20 to 25 cycles per minute

11. What is the recommended gait where a patient has one weight bearing leg?

    a. Four-point gait
    b. Three-point gait
    c. Two-point gait
    d. Swing-to gait

12. What is the gait where a patient moves one crutch forward and the opposite leg?

    a. Three-point gait
    b. Swing-to gait
    c. Four-point gait
    d. Two-point gait

13. Hot-to-cold plunges are examples of:

    a. Hydrotherapy
    b. Cryotherapy
    c. Thermotherapy
    d. None of the Above

14. What type of crutches are used for long-term disability?

    a. Standard crutches
    b. Auxillary crutches
    c. Lofstrand crutches
    d. None of the Above

15. Which of the following is the correct fitting for crutch hand grips?

    a. Adjust hand grips to 30 degrees of elbow flexion
    b. Adjust hand grips to 45 degrees of elbow flexion
    c. Adjust hand grips to 20 degrees of elbow flexion
    d. Adjust hand grips to 25 degrees of elbow flexion

16. Which type of passive exercise is typically used to alleviate pain and improve function?

    a. Passive motion
    b. Massage
    c. Electrical stimulation
    d. None of the Above

17. What is the correct way to fit a walker for a patient?

    a. With elbow straight
    b. With elbow flexed at 30 degrees
    c. With elbow flexed at 20 degrees
    d. With elbow flexed at 45 degrees

18. What are standard precautions when a patient is getting out of a wheelchair?

    a. Lock wheels and place patient's arms around your neck
    b. Lock wheels and do not allow patient's arms around your neck
    c. Lock wheels and do not allow patient's arms around your neck
    d. None of the Above

Section III – Clinical Pharmacology

19. What type of drug is commonly used for decreasing a cough?

    a. Antiemetic
    b. Antihypertensive
    c. Antitussive
    d. Decongestant

20. Celebrex is commonly used for

    a. Decreasing fever
    b. decreasing diarrhea
    c. Dilating the bronchi
    d. Decreasing inflammation

21. Which of the following is commonly used as an antihypertensive?

    a. Compazine
    b. Lopressor
    c. Heparin
    d. Ibuprofen

22. A drug that is injected into the skin is called

    a. Intradermal
    b. Interdermal
    c. Intramuscular
    d. Intermuscula

23. What are drops placed in the ear called?

    a. Optic
    b. Oral
    c. Otic
    d. Ophthalmic

Section IV – Minor Surgery

24. Identify the instrument below

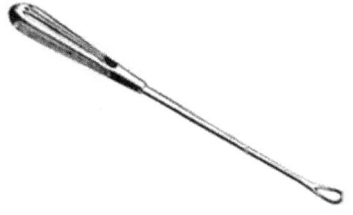

   a. Needle Holder
   b. Tenaculum
   c. Curettes
   d. Hemostats

25. Identify the instrument below:

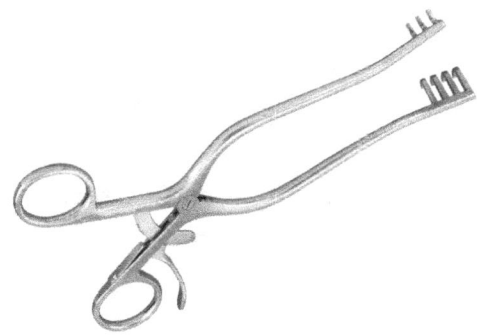

   a. Tenaculum
   b. Probe
   c. Curettes
   d. Retractors

26. Identify the instrument below:

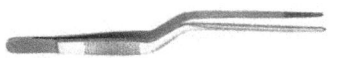

a. Probe
b. Retractors
c. Bayonet forceps
d. Tenaculum

27. Identify the instrument below:

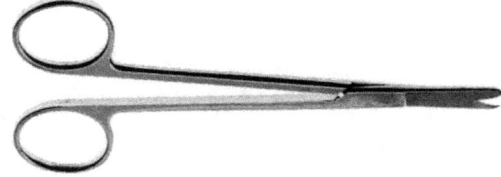

a. Bandage scissors
b. Surgical scissors
c. Suture removal scissors
d. Tenaculum

28. Which of the following is not a guideline for sterile fields?

a. Allow only sterile items to come into contact with other sterile items.

b. Do not leave the sterile field unattended for more than 5 minutes.

c. Maintain a border of 1 inch between the sterile field and non-sterile area.

d. Do not pass contaminated items over a sterile field.

29. A sterile saline liquid must be transferred to a sterile waterproof container. How should this be done?

    a. Over the sterile field.

    b. Beside the sterile field.

    c. Away from the sterile field.

    d. The sterile container should not touch the sterile field.

Section V – Lab and ECG

30. What is collected in a collection tube with a lavender top?

    a. Plasma for urgent chemical testing

    b. Blood for glucose testing

    c. Plasma for haematology testing

    d. Serum for chemical testing

31. What is collected in a collection tube with a red top?

    a. Serum for chemical testing

    b. Plasma for haematology testing

    c. Plasma for urgent chemical testing

    d. Serum for chemistry and serology

32. What is the correct order of collection for collection tubes?

    a. Yellow, Red, Lavender, Speckled, Blue, Green, Gray

    b. Yellow, Red, Speckled, Lavender, Blue, Green, Gray

    c. Yellow, Speckled, Lavender, Red, Blue, Green, Gray

    d. Red, Yellow, Speckled, Lavender, Blue, Green, Gray

33. What is a common specimen collected from a lumbar puncture?

   a. Biopsy

   b. Urethral brushings

   c. Cerebral spinal fluid

   d. None of the Above

34. What is the difference between a random and a first voided urine sample?

   a. A random sample is anytime and a first voided is collected in the morning

   b. A random sample is collected over a 24 hour period and a first voided is collected first thing in the morning

   c. A first voided sample is collected anytime and a random sample is collected first thing in the morning.

   d. None of the Above

35. What is a postprandial sample?

   a. Collect first thing in the morning

   b. Collected after the patient has eaten

   c. Collected after the patient has drank two large glasses of water

   d. Collected mid-stream

36. What is an evacuated tube?

   a. A collection tube that is empty

   b. A collection tube that has been emptied

   c. A collection tube with a lavender top

   d. A sealed collection tube

37. What is fibrinogen?

   a. An additive to collection tubes
   b. A protein that assists clotting
   c. Abnormal blood cells
   d. None of the Above

38. What is human chorionic gonadotropin?

   a. A hormone present during pregnancy
   b. A disease causing physical and mental handicaps
   c. A protein that assists clotting
   d. A type of antibody

39. What is a heart rate shorter than 60 bpm called?

   a. Tachycardia
   b. Asystole
   c. Bradycardia
   d. Ectopic beat

40. What is a heart rate faster than 100 bpm called?

   a. Bradycardia
   b. Tachycardia
   c. Bigeminy
   d. Asystole

41. What is a premature ventricular tachycardia?

   a. Early contraction of the ventricles
   b. A ventricular rate of more than 100 to 150 bpm
   c. Ventricular fibrillation
   d. Uncoordinated ventricular contractrions

42. What is a ventricular flutter?

    a. Ventricular rate of 100 to 150 bpm
    b. Ventricular rate of 60 - 100 bpm
    c. A ventricular rate of 150 to 300 bpm
    d. Uncoordinated ventricular contractions

43. What is a possible cause of a wandering baseline?

    a. Leads are too tight or too loose
    b. Patient is moving around
    c. ECG machine malfunction
    d. Electrodes too loose or too tight

44. What is a possible cause of an interrupted baseline?

    a. patient moving
    b. patient wearing lotion
    c. a wire coming disconnected
    d. hot or sluggish stylus

45. What type of test used sound waves to test for abnormalities?

    a. Echocardiogram
    b. Halter monitor
    c. Angiogram
    d. Cardiac catheterization

Answer Key

1. D
Osteoporosis is a disease of bones that leads to an increased risk of fracture.

2. D
Marfan syndrome (also called Marfan's syndrome) is a genetic disorder of the connective tissue.

3. D
The circulatory system can be thought of as the blood distribution system.

4. B
The circulatory system is responsible for passing gases, blood cells, hormones, and nutrients, like electrolytes and amino acids, to and from the various groups of cells in the body, fight off diseases, and stabilize both the pH level and body temperature to maintain a level of homeostasis that is vital to proper function.

5. C
The organ system responsible for transporting nutrients, hormones, blood cells, nutrients, etc in and out of the body's cells in an effort to stabilize body temperature, pH levels, fight off diseases, and ensure homeostasis is known as the circulatory system.

6. A
The main components of the circulatory system are the heart, veins and blood vessels.

7. D
The circulatory system disease that is one of the most frequent causes of death in North America is heart disease.

8. C
Angina is a condition that is often assumed to actually be a heart attack. More accurately known as angina pectoris, this is cause by ischemia, or a lack of blood flowing into the heart muscle and, as a result oxygen. It is often the result of

obstructions, or spasms, of blood vessels in the heart.

9. B
High blood pressure is a more common name for the circulatory system disease known as hypertension. Hypertension (HTN) or high blood pressure is a cardiac chronic medical condition in which the systemic arterial blood pressure is elevated.

10. D
The term cardiac dysrhythmia, sometimes known as irregular heartbeat or arrhythmia, refers to any of the conditions that fit the large and heterogeneous groups that involve abnormal electrical activity inside the human heart. This can be a heartbeat that is too fast, too slow, regular, or irregular.

11. A
The anatomical system, inside any organism, that is responsible for introducing gases to the body's interior and exchanging it is known as the respiratory system. The respiratory system features anatomical features such as lungs, airways, and respiratory muscles. Carbon dioxide and oxygen molecules are taken in and exchanged between the blood and the environment by a process of diffusion. More specifically, this process of exchange takes place in the alveolar region in the lungs.

12. B
The lungs are an important component of the respiratory system.

13. D
The exchange of oxygen for carbon dioxide takes place in the alveolar area of the lungs.

14. B
The thoracic diaphragm, is a sheet of internal skeletal muscle that extends across the bottom of the rib cage. The diaphragm performs an important function in respiration.

15. A
Exhalation is often accomplished by the abdominal muscles.

Practice Test Questions Set 2

16. D
The blood is the primary thing oxygenated through the work of the respiratory system.

17. C
An important side-benefit of the respiratory system is the air being expelled from the mouth allows for speaking.

18. A
Emphysema is a long-term, progressive disease of the lungs that primarily causes shortness of breath.

19. C
The immune system is the system that protects the body from disease and infection.

20. A
The immune system fights off disease by identifying and killing tumor cells and pathogens.

21. D
An example of a pathogen that the immune system detects is A virus.

22. A
Detection of pathogens can be complicated because they evolve so quickly.

23. B
One of the best-known disorders that attack the immune system is HIV (the virus that causes AIDS).

24. A
The process by which the immune system adapts over time to be more efficient in recognizing pathogens is known as acquired immunity.

25. B
Inflammation is an example of an early response by the immune system to infection.

26. B
White blood cells are an important weapon in the fight

against infection.

27. D
The primary purpose of the digestive system is to convert food into a form that can provide nourishment for the body.

28. A
Gastric acid is a digestive fluid, formed in the stomach. It has a pH of 1 to 2 and is composed of hydrochloric acid and large quantities of potassium chloride and sodium chloride.

29. D
Digestion begins in the mouth.

30. B
Cleansing food of impurities is not an example of a function of the stomach in digestion.

31. A
Fats stay in the stomach longest.

32. C
Indigestion is a common digestive affliction that most people suffer at one time or other.

33. B
Diverticulitis is a pouch in the large intestine becomes inflamed.

34. A
Eating a healthy diet is the best way to avoid most digestive diseases.

35. D
Producing, storing and eliminating urine are the three functions of the urinary system.

36. B
Urine is mostly comprised of waste material after the body has taken the nutrients from food and absorbed the water it needs.

37. A
Urea is the name of the waste removed from the body through urine.

38. B
Carrying urea to the kidneys is one example of the blood stream's part in the digestive system.

39. D
Besides the kidney, the other major organ that takes part in the body's urinary system is the Bladder

40. B
The bladder is a balloon shaped, muscular organ.

41. C
Kidney failure is an example of one of the many serious urinary disorders.

42. A
The involuntary passage of urine defines the urinary-system disorder known as incontinence.

43. A
The lymphatic system is the system which carries a clear liquid lymph toward the heart.

44. B
Lymphoid tissue exists in many organs, although it's predominantly in the lymph nodes.

45. C
An example of an organ that plays a big role in the lymphatic system is the spleen.

46. D
Among the benefits of the lymphatic system is the fact that it Absorbs and transports fats and fatty acids from the body's circulatory system.

47. A
Metastasis is a process of carrying cancer cells between various parts of the body.

48. B
A common affliction of the lymphatic system is swelling of the lymph nodes.

49. A
An example of a cause of lymph node swelling is Infectious mononucleosis ("Mono").

50. D
Another, more serious, example of a cause of lymph node swelling is Cancer.

Section II – Medical Terminology

1. A
Bodily organs can sometimes adhere to the peritoneum, a two-layered membrane lining the abdominal cavity and covering abdominal organs; when this occurs, it the problem is corrected through surgical release of peritoneal adhesions.

2. C
A/an biopsy allows a physician to obtain a small, representative sample of tissue for microscopic examination; this is usually done to establish a diagnosis.

3. A
Inguinal hernia repair is indicated when part of the intestine protrudes into the groin.

4. C
Hemorrhoids are distended veins in the lower rectum or anus; a hemorrhoidectomy is performed to relieve this condition.

5. B
During open carpal tunnel surgery, a tight band of transverse fibrous tissue is cut, releasing pressure on the median nerves and relieving symptoms.

6. A
A surgical procedure that unblocks the arteries located in the neck which supply blood to the brain is a/an Carotid endarterectomy.

Practice Test Questions Set 2   175

7. D
Cataract surgery involves removal of the opaque contents of a lens of the eye via ultrasound waves, although, in some cases, the entire lens is removed and replaced with an artificial lens.

8. C
Following a radical hysterectomy, a small number of patients are placed on a hormone replacement regimen.

9. C
The following statement is false: Fluoroscopy produces a series of still images of the body part being examined.

10. A
A/an angiogram is a test employed to identify blockages in the circulatory system, diagnose stroke and determine the size and location of brain tumors and aneurysms.

11. B
During a biopsy, a small sample of tissue is removed, usually under local anesthetic, examined microscopically for diagnosis.

12. A
Electromyography (EMG) is a technique for evaluating and recording the electrical activity produced by skeletal muscles.

13. B
The following statement about cerebrospinal fluid analysis is false: A lumbar puncture is performed to obtain a fluid sample, a painless procedure completed without the use of anesthetic.

14. D
Computed tomography, also known as a CT scan, is used to detect bone and vascular anomalies, certain types of brain tumors, and blood clots in patients who have experienced a stroke or brain damage due to an injury.

15. D
Using the magnetic properties of the blood, a Functional MRI

(fMRI) produces real-time images of blood flow to certain areas of the brain and assesses damage due to head injury or disorders such as Alzheimer's disease.

16. C
The following statement is false, PET scans are frequently used instead of CT or MRI scans, which are significantly less accurate.

17. B
Physiatry and rehabilitation medicine, or PM&R, is a branch of medical practice that has the goal of restoring and enhancing the quality of life and functional ability of patients who are living with disabilities or impairments. A physiatrist or rehab medicine specialist is a physician who has gone through all the proper field work as part of their physician training. Physiatrists are specialists in restoring function to their patients when they must live with injuries to the nervous system, for stroke patients, but also injuries to tissues, bones, and muscles.

18. D
Colorectal surgery is a field in medicine, dealing with disorders of the rectum, anus, and colon. Proctology is the most commonly used name for this field of medicine. The physicians who specialize in these types of procedures are known as proctologists or colorectal surgeons.

19. D
Pulmonology (AKA pneumology or respirology) is the specialty that deals with diseases of the respiratory tract and respiratory disease. Some regions and countries refer to this field as respiratory medicine or chest medicine. It is closely related to intensive care medicine, although pulmonology is more commonly considered to be a part of internal medicine. The classification with intensive care medicine is usually due to the treatment of patients who require ventilation through mechanical means. However, chest medicine isn't a specialty on its own, as it is simply an inclusive term that covers a variety of treatments, including diseases inside of the chest and also includes pulmonology, intensive care medicine, and thoracic surgery.

20. B
Rheumatology is a sub-specialty in internal medicine and pediatrics, devoted to diagnosis and therapy of rheumatic diseases. Rheumatologists are physicians who specialize in this particular field. As a rheumatologist, these physicians treat several clinical problems that can involve autoimmune diseases, soft tissues, joints, vasculitis, and heritable connective tissue disorders as well.

21. A
Vascular medicine, known in Europe as angiology, is a medical specialty centered on the study of the circulatory and lymphatic systems and diseases associated with those systems.

22. D
All for the statements are true.

> Thoracic surgeons treat diseases that affect the organs within the chest.
> Treatment most frequently involves conditions of the lungs, chest wall and diaphragm.
> Many times, thoracic surgery is grouped with cardiac surgery and termed cardio-thoracic surgery.

23. B
The surgical and medical specialty of Urology is focused on treating problems in males and females' urinary tracts and the male reproductive system. Those who specialize in this medical field are called urologists and have been trained to treat, diagnose, and then manage patients who have disorders in their urological systems. Several organs are involved and can include ureters, adrenal glands, kidneys, urethra, and the organs of the male reproductive system, like the seminal vesicles, penis, prostate, vas deferens, testes, and epididymis. For physicians entering the field, this can be one of the most competitive.

24. C
Cardiac surgeons are responsible for performing cardiovascular surgeries involving the heart and the heart's vessels. This is commonly done to treat medical complications associated with ischemic heart disease, such as coronary artery

bypass grafting, treat valvular heart diseases, or correct problems with congenital heart disease. These can be caused by atherosclerosis, rheumatic heart disease, or endocarditis. Cardiovascular surgeons are also responsible for complicated heart transplants.

Section III – Medical Law and Ethics

1. C
In many U.S. states and Australia, **mandated reporters** are professionals who, in the ordinary course of their work and because they have regular contact with children, disabled persons, senior citizens, or other identified vulnerable populations, are required to report (or cause a report to be made) whenever financial, physical, sexual or other types of abuse has been observed or is suspected, or when there is evidence of neglect, knowledge of an incident, or an imminent risk of serious harm. For example, in South Australia, a school teacher must report a child attending school seeming malnourished or presenting with bruising, complaining of neglect or otherwise demonstrating neglect or abuse at home, to child welfare authorities.

These professionals can be held liable by both the civil and criminal legal systems for intentionally failing to make a report but their name can also be said unidentified. Mandated reporters also include persons who have assumed full or intermittent responsibility for the care or custody of a child, dependent adult, or elder, whether or not they are compensated for their services. RAINN maintains a database of mandatory reporting regulations regarding children and the elderly by state, including who is required to report, standards of knowledge, definitions of a victim, to whom the report must be made, information required in the report, and regulations regarding timing and other procedures. [11]

2. A
Signs of physical child abuse may include but are not limited to:
- Inability to recall how injuries occurred or offers an inconsistent explanation
- wary of adults

- may cringe or flinch if touched unexpectedly
- infants may display a vacant stare
- extremely aggressive or extremely withdrawn
- indiscriminately seeks affection
- extremely compliant and/or eager to please

3. A
Signs of emotional abuse may include but are not limited to:

- severe depression
- Non-attachment to the parent
- extreme withdrawal or aggressiveness
- overly compliant, too well mannered, too neat or clean
- extreme attention seeking
- displays extreme inhibition in play

4. D
Signs of sexual abuse may include but are not limited to:

- age inappropriate play with toys, self or others displaying explicit sexual acts
- age inappropriate sexually explicit drawing and/or descriptions
- bizarre, sophisticated or unusual sexual knowledge
- prostitution
- seductive behaviors

5. D
Child neglect is defined as:

- "the failure of a person responsible for a child's care and upbringing to safeguard the child's emotional and physical health and general well-being"
- acts of commission, harm to a child may or may not be the intended consequence
- a serious form of maltreatment
- the persistent failure to meet a child's basic physical and/or psychological needs resulting in serious impairment of health and/or development.

6. D
All the following are signs of fetal abuse:

- Poor fetal growth on abdomen measurements or ultrasound
- History or signs of domestic abuse
- History or signs of maternal alcohol or drug use

7. D
The following statements are used by the Uniform Determination of Death Act (UDDA) to define death

- The individual has sustained irreversible cessation of circulatory and respiratory functions.
- The individual has sustained irreversible cessation of all functions of the entire brain, including the brain stem.

8. B
Malfeasance is also known as misfeasance and nonfeasance.

9. C
Government agencies such as Medicare, Workers Compensation and Social Security Disability Insurance

10. A
The medical information of a person at risk for HIV being released without patient permission in an emergency situation to medical personnel or a court order has been issued.

11. B
Distributive justice refers to what society owes a person in proportion to their individual needs and responsibilities, the resources available and society's responsibilities to the common good.

12. A
The term managed care is used in the United States to describe a variety of techniques intended to reduce the cost of providing health benefits and improve the quality of care ("managed care techniques") for organizations that use those techniques or provide them as services to other organizations ("managed care organization" or "MCO"), or to describe systems of financing and delivering health care to enrollees organized around managed care techniques and concepts ("managed care delivery systems"). According to the United

States National Library of Medicine, the term "managed care" encompasses programs:

...intended to reduce unnecessary health care costs through a variety of mechanisms, including: economic incentives for physicians and patients to select less costly forms of care; programs for reviewing the medical necessity of specific services; increased beneficiary cost sharing; controls on inpatient admissions and lengths of stay; the establishment of cost-sharing incentives for outpatient surgery; selective contracting with health care providers; and the intensive management of high-cost health care cases. The programs may be provided in a variety of settings, such as Health Maintenance Organizations and Preferred Provider Organizations. [12]

13. B
Benefits available to immigrants include school lunch and breakfast programs, immunizations, emergency medical services, disaster relief, and others programs that are necessary to protect life and safety as identified by the attorney general, regardless of immigration status

14. C
A Do Not Resuscitate (DNR) indicates that a patient does not want cardiopulmonary resuscitation or defibrillation at the end of life, while a DNI order indicates that the patient rejects the use of a breathing tube in cases of respiratory arrest. Both can be revoked at any time.

15. C
In American law, competence concerns the mental capacity of an individual to participate in legal proceedings.

16. B
Civil law, as opposed to criminal law, is the branch of law dealing with disputes between individuals or organizations, in which compensation may be awarded to the victim. For instance, if a car crash victim claims damages against the driver for loss or injury sustained in an accident, this will be a civil law case.

17. D
Cultural competence refers to an ability to interact effectively with people of different cultures.

The term cultural competence specifically refers to a person's ability to effectively communicate with patients of a wide range of cultures and backgrounds, most commonly in the context of non-profit organizations, human resources, or government groups who have employees that are diverse and come from a number of different ethnic backgrounds.

There are four components of this ability:

> 1) A knowledge of a person's own world view in regards to their culture
> 2) An open attitude in regard to cultural differences
> 3) An understanding of varying worldviews and cultural practices
> 4) Skills to allow cross-cultural communication. The development of these skills is vital to communicating, understanding, and effectively treating people who are of different cultural backgrounds.

18. A
A 2006 follow-up to the 2000 Institute of Medicine study found that medication errors are among the most common medical mistakes, harming at least 1.5 million people every year. According to the study, 400,000 preventable drug-related injuries occur each year in hospitals, 800,000 in long-term care settings, and roughly 530,000 among Medicare recipients in outpatient clinics. The report stated that these are likely to be conservative estimates. In 2000 alone, the extra medical costs incurred by preventable drug related injuries approximated $887 million — and the study looked only at injuries sustained by Medicare recipients, a subset of clinic visitors. None of these figures take into account lost wages and productivity or other costs.

According to a 2002 Agency for Healthcare Research and Quality report, about 7,000 people were estimated to die each year from medication errors - about 16 percent more deaths than the number attributable to work-related injuries (6,000 deaths) [13]

19. D
Types of medication errors include:

- Administration errors which occur when the provider gives the wrong medicine to the patient
- Pharmacy fulfillment errors
- Transcription errors which occur when the pharmacist misreads the prescription or it is written incorrectly

20. A
The law demands that patients are treated compassionately, while ethics require competent medical practice according to current standards and frequently exceed legal standards.

21. D
A medical professional cannot refuse to treat a patient with an infectious disease.

22. C
The Health Insurance Portability and Accountability Act of 1996 was enacted by the U.S. Congress and signed by President Bill Clinton in 1996.

23. C
Adolescents must always obtain parental permission before placing a child for adoption.

24. A
An emancipated minor is a minor who is allowed to conduct a business or any other occupation on his or her own behalf or for their own account outside the influence of a parent or guardian.

25. A
A fiduciary duty is a legal or ethical relationship of confidence or trust between two or more parties. Typically, a fiduciary prudently takes care of money for another person.

Section IV – Communication Skills and Patient Education

1. B
Level of education can act as a barrier to communication.

2. A
Personal space is the zone around each person reserved for conversation and can vary according to culture.

3. D
When dealing with elderly patients, always address them as Miss, Mrs., or Mr., followed by their last name.

4. B
A complete medical history should include the chief complaint.

5. C
When documenting a patient's chief complaint, be careful to use the patient's exact words.

6. D
Physical barriers to communication include, time, environment, and illness.

7. A
If a patient does not seem to understand a question, repeat the question using simpler terms. Asking if they understand or skipping the question are not helpful.

8. D
Perception checking is repeating what someone has said to check the accuracy of the information.

9. C
For patients who are depressed, with cognitive impairment, or unable to deal with complex communication at that particular moment, using direct questions that require short answers can help obtain information.

Practice Test Questions Set 2

10. B
Silence should always be avoided in the interview process is false. Silence can be very useful during an interview, as it can allow patients to think about their answer.

11. C
A leading question is a question that suggests the answer.

12. A
Leading questions are an ineffective means of obtaining information because the patient may feel forced to give the answer the interviewer is looking for.

13. D
During the interview process, the most accurate information is provided by the patient.

14. A
When interviewing a patient with a hearing loss, remember to Speak slowly and look directly at the patient.

15. D
The medical record is the key means of communication between healthcare workers.

16. B
A health history is used to obtain subjective information and learn about past and current health problems.

17. C
Biographical information is the first area to be covered when obtaining a health history.

18. C
Using neutral remarks such as, "I see" and "I hear what you're saying" shows understanding to the patient.

19. D
Besides providing accurate patient information to other healthcare professionals, it is necessary that one be able to interpret what others have added to the medical record.

20. A
If a patient refuses to make eye contact, you may find that they are from a culture that considers direct eye contact rude.

Part II – Administrative Medical Assisting

Section I – Insurance Answer Key

1. B
The Birthday Rule is where a person is covered by two insurance policies. The policy to be billed is determined by the policyholder whose birthday comes first in the calendar year.

2. C
Workers' Compensation is a form of insurance providing wage replacement and medical benefits to employees injured in the course of employment in exchange for mandatory relinquishment of the employee's right to sue his or her employer for the tort of negligence. The trade-off between assured, limited coverage and lack of recourse outside the worker compensation system is known as "the compensation bargain." [5]

3. D
AN EOB, also called remittance advice, is an explanation of what is covered and what is not covered and why.

4. A
Some insurance companies use a method called, Usual, Customary and Reasonable that compares Physician's charges for a procedure in a geographical area.

5. B
Pre-certification, also known as pre-authorization. Most insurance companies require pre-certification 24 hours before a patient is admitted or undergoes certain procedures.

6. A
Usual, Customary and Reasonable is also called the Prevailing Fee.

7. A
An Indemnity Plan is a health insurance plan where all or a part of the costs are covered, for any physician, hospital or licensed provider.

8. C
Starting in 1997, Medicare beneficiaries were given the option to receive their Medicare benefits through private health insurance plans, instead of through the original Medicare plan (Parts A and B). These programs were known as "Medicare+Choice" or "Part C" plans.

9. A
Assignment of benefits authorizes payment to be sent to the provider. In fact, the assignment of benefits is the transfer of the patient's legal right to collect benefits to the provider.

10. B
Relative Value Studies list the procedure codes and relative values, allowing a comparison of costs for the different codes.

11. A
Co-payment, also called coinsurance, is the cost or percentage the insured person pays.

12. A
Diagnosis-related group (DRG) is a system to classify hospital cases into one of originally 467 groups. The 467th was "Ungroupable." The system is also called "the DRGs," and its intent was to identify the "products" that a hospital provides. One example of a "product" is an appendectomy. The system was developed at Yale, in anticipation of convincing Congress to use it for reimbursement, to replace "cost based" reimbursement that was used up to that point. DRGs are assigned by a "grouper" program based on ICD (International Classification of Diseases) diagnoses, procedures, age, sex, discharge status, and the presence of complications or comorbidities. DRGs have been used in the US since 1982

to determine how much Medicare pays the hospital for each "product," since patients within each category are similar clinically and are expected to use the same level of hospital resources. DRGs may be further grouped into Major Diagnostic Categories (MDCs).

13. D
Pre-certification, also knows as pre-authorization. Most insurance companies require Pre-certification 24 hours before a patient is admitted or undergoes certain procedures.

14. A
A Third-Party Payer is who ever pays the doctor or hospital for services, usually a public or private insurance company.

Section II – Coding and Claims

15. A
Unbundling is the process where several CPT codes are used for a procedure that is normally covered by one code.

16. D
CPT Codes for Surgery: 10021-69990

(10021 - 10022) general
(10040 - 19499) integumentary system
(20000 - 29999) musculoskeletal system
(30000 - 32999) respiratory system
(33010 - 37799) cardiovascular system
(38100 - 38999) hemic & lymphatic systems
(39000 - 39599) mediastinum & diaphragm
(40490 - 49999) digestive system
(50010 - 53899) urinary system
(54000 - 55899) male genital system
(55920 - 55980) reproductive system & intersex
(56405 - 58999) female genital system
(59000 - 59899) maternity care & delivery
(60000 - 60699) endocrine system
(61000 - 64999) nervous system
(65091 - 68899) eye & ocular adnexa
(69000 - 69979) auditory system

17. C
ICD-9 V codes identify health care visits for reasons other than illness.
ICD-9 E codes identifies the cause of injury and mechanism of injury.
ICD-9 S codes do not exist.

18. A
Dirty Claims are claims rejected by the insurance company due to errors or other reasons.

19. B
Split billing is billing for several visits when only one visit occurred.

20. C
The CMS-1500 is the Universal Claim Form. Historically, claims were submitted using a paper form; for professional (non-hospital) services and for most payers the CMS-1500 form or HCFA (Health Care Financing Administration claim form) was commonly used. The CMS-1500 form is so named for its originator, the Centers for Medicare and Medicaid Services. At time of writing, about 30% of medical claims are sent to payers using paper forms that are either manually entered or entered using automated recognition or OCR software.

Claims are usually filed electronically by formatting the claim as an ANSI 837 file and using Electronic Data Interchange to submit the claim file to the payer directly or via a clearinghouse. [14]

21. C
Etiology is the study of causation, or origination.

22. C
J-codes (example: J0120): Drugs Administered Other Than Oral Method, Chemotherapy Drugs

23. A
G-codes (example: G0008): Temporary Procedures & Professional Services

24. A
ICD-9 E codes identifies the cause of injury and mechanism of injury.

Section III – Finance and Bookkeeping

25. D
Accounts receivable represents money owed by entities to the firm on the sale of products or services on credit

26. A
An adjustment in accounting is a change to the amount owed for reasons other than payments or changes in services, such as a refund or discount.

27. C
The Accounts Receivable Age Analysis Printout monitors all of the Accounts Receivable accounts that a company has. This is called the Debtors Book and can be divided into different categories depending on their current status and the length of time that they have been overdue. Modern Accounting System produces these and are organized in the order set by the Chart of Accounts for the Debtors Book.

28. B
Accounts payable are a Liability for the business.

29. B
A customer check returned by the bank will be marked NSF for Not Sufficient Funds.

30. B
To endorse a check is to sign the back.

31. B
Tax withheld for Social Security and Medicare is called the Federal Insurance and Contribution Act (FICA).

32. B
A purchase order is sent to the supplier by the medical office.

33. C
An adjustment in accounting is a change to the amount owed for reasons other than payments or changes in services, such as a refund or discount.

34. B
Checks that you aren't going to use should be marked Void, to prevent use by unauthorized persons.

Part III – Clinical Medical Assisting

Section I – Asepsis

1. C
The United States Occupational Safety and Health Administration (OSHA) is an agency of the United States Department of Labor. Its mission is to prevent work-related injuries, illnesses, and occupational fatality by issuing and enforcing standards for workplace safety and health.

2. D
A person with normal immunity is not considered a susceptible host.

3. C
To ensure the autoclave has finished sterilizing, both the pressure gauge and the time should be zero.

4. A
The most important standard precaution is to treat all bodily fluids as contaminated.

5. B
A Hospital Acquired Infection, also known as HAI or a nosocomial infection, is a unique type of infection. These favor the environment of a hospital and a patient can acquire them while they are staying there, or it can infect hospital staff while they are working. These bacterial and fungal infections take advantage of the hospital patient's impaired immune system.

6. C
Influenza, commonly called the flu, is an infectious disease caused by RNA viruses of the family Orthomyxoviridae (the influenza viruses), that affects birds and mammals.

7. B
A pathogen is any infectious agent. Lichen are not an infectious agent.

Section II – Vital Signs and Physical Modalities

8. D
60 to 100 bpm is the normal adult pulse.

9. A
Circulation to the extremities is usually measured at the Popliteal artery just above the knee.

10. B
12 to 20 cycles per minute is the normal respiration rate for an adult.

11. B
3-point gait sequence is first move both crutches and the weaker lower limb forward. Then bear all your weight down through the crutches, and move the stronger leg forward.

The 3-point gait eliminates all weight bearing on the affected leg.

12. D
The two-point crutch gait is used when there is weakness in both legs or poor coordination.

The sequence is left crutch and right foot together, then the right crutch and left foot together.

13. A
Hydrotherapy, formerly called hydropathy, involves the use of water for pain-relief and treating illness.

Practice Test Questions Set 2

14. C
Forearm crutches are crutches with a cuff at the top to go around the forearm, and are also known as the Lofstrand crutch.

15. A
The correct fitting for crutch handgrips is to adjust handgrips to 30 degrees of elbow flexion.

16. B
Massage is a passive exercise is typically used to alleviate pain and improve function.

17. B
The correct way to fit a walker for a patient is with elbow flexed at 30 degrees.

18. B
Standard precautions when a patient is getting out of a wheelchair is to lock the wheels and do not allow patient's arms around your neck.

Section III –Clinical Pharmacology

19. C
A cough medicine (or linctus, when in syrup form) is a medicinal drug used in an attempt to treat coughing and related conditions.

20. D
Celecoxib is a sulfa non-steroidal anti-inflammatory drug (NSAID) and selective COX-2 inhibitor used in the treatment of osteoarthritis, rheumatoid arthritis, acute pain, painful menstruation and menstrual symptoms, and to reduce numbers of colon and rectum polyps in patients with familial adenomatous polyposis. It is marketed by Pfizer. It is known under the brand name Celebrex or Celebra for arthritis and Onsenal for polyps.

21. B
Metoprolol is a selective β1 receptor blocker used in treatment of several diseases of the cardiovascular system, es-

pecially hypertension. It is marketed under the brand name Lopressor by Novartis.

22. A
Intradermal means between layers of skin.

23. C
Otic means of, or relating to the ear.

Section IV – Minor Surgery

24. C
A curette is a surgical instrument designed for scraping biological tissue or debris in a biopsy, excision, or cleaning procedure.

25. D
A retractor is a surgical instrument by which a surgeon can either actively separate the edges of a surgical incision or wound, or can hold back underlying organs and tissues, so that body parts under the incision may be accessed.

26. C
Bayonet forceps

27. C
Suture removal scissors

28. B
Leaving a sterile field un-attended for any length of time is NOT a guideline. Sterile fields should be attended at all times.

29. A
Always transfer sterile materials to sterile containers over the sterile field.

Section V – Lab and ECG

30. C
Plasma for hematology testing is collected in a Lavender top

collection tube.

31. D
Serum for chemistry and serology is collected in a red top collection tube.

32. B
The correct order is Yellow, Red, Speckled, Lavender, Blue, Green, Gray.

33. C
A lumbar puncture (or LP, and colloquially known as a spinal tap) is a diagnostic and at times therapeutic procedure that is performed to collect a sample of cerebrospinal fluid (CSF).

34. A
A random sample is anytime and a first voided is collected in the morning.

35. B
A postprandial sample is a sample taken after eating.

36. D
An evacuated tube is a sealed collection tube.

37. B
Fibrinogen (factor I) is a soluble plasma glycoprotein, synthesised by the liver, that is converted by thrombin into fibrin during blood coagulation.

38. A
Human chorionic gonadotropin or human chorionic gonadotrophin (hCG) is a glycoprotein hormone produced during.

39. C
Bradycardia is the resting heart rate of fewer than 60 beats per minute, though it is seldom symptomatic until the rate drops below 50 beat/min.

40. B
Tachycardia typically refers to a heart rate that exceeds the normal range.

41. B
Ventricular tachycardia (V-tach or VT) is a tachycardia, or fast heart rhythm, that originates in one of the ventricles of the heart.

42. C
Ventricular flutter is an arrhythmia, more specifically a tachycardia affecting the ventricles with a rate over 200 beats/min.

43. D
A wandering baseline is where the stylus moves from the center in a 'wandering' fashion, often caused by too tight or too lose electrodes.

44. C
A broken baseline, as the name implies is a break between complexes, usually caused by a disconnection.

45. A
An echocardiogram, often called, in the medical community, a cardiac ECHO, is a sonogram of the heart.

Pharmacy Dosage Problems

1. The physician orders 40 mg Depo-Medrol; 80 mg/mL is on hand. How many milliliters are required?

    a. 0.5 ml
    b. 0.80 ml
    c. 0.25 ml
    d. 0.40 ml

2. The physician orders 750 mg Tagamet liquid; 1500 mg/tsp is on hand. How many teaspoons are required?

    a. 0.75 tsp
    b. 0.5 tsp
    c. 1 tsp
    d. 2 tsp

3. The physician ordered 75 mg of Seconal; 50 mg/mL is on hand. How many mL are required?

    a. 2 mL
    b. 1 mL
    c. 1.5 ml
    d. .5 mL

4. The physician ordered 1,500 mg Duricef; 1g/tablet is on hand. How many tablets are required?

    a. 1 Tablet
    b. 1.5 Tables
    c. 2 Tablets
    d. None of the Above.

5. The physician orders 150 mg morphine sulphate; 1 g/mL is on hand. How many mL are required?

a. 0.25 mL
b. 0.15 mL
c. 0.50 mL
d. 0.35 mL

6. The physician ordered 10 units of regular insulin; 100 U/mL is on hand. How many milliliters are required?

a. 1.0 mL
b. 0.5 mL
c. 0.01 mL
d. 0.1 mL

7. The physician ordered 5 mg Coumadin; 5 mg/tablet is on hand. How many tablets are required?

a. 0.5 tablets
b. 1 tablet
c. 1.5 tablets
d. .25 tablets

8. The physician ordered 20 mg Tylenol/kg of body weight; on hand is 80 mg/tablet. The child weighs 12 kg. How many tablets are required?

a. 3 tablets
b. 1 tablet
c. 1.5 tablets
d. .5 tablets

Pharmacy Dosage Problems

9. The physician ordered 20 mg Tylenol/kg of body weight; on hand is 80 mg/tablet. The child weighs 44 lb. How many tablets are required?

   a. 5 tablets
   b. 4 tablets
   c. 7 tablets
   d. 2 tablets

10. The physician ordered 3,000 units of heparin and 5,000 U/mL is on hand. How many milliliters are required?

    a. 1 mL
    b. 0.5 mL
    c. .06 mL
    d. 0.6 mL

11. The physician orders 60 mg Augmentin; 80 mg/mL is on hand. How many milliliters are required?

    a. 1 mL
    b. 0.75 mL
    c. 0.5 mL
    d. 1.5 mL

12. The physician ordered 16 mg Ibuprofen/kg of body weight; on hand is 80 mg/tablet. The child weighs 15 kg. How many tablets are required?

    a. 1 Tablet
    b. 2 Tablets
    c. 3 Tablets
    d. 4 Tablets

13. The physician orders 1000 mg Benadryl liquid; 1 g/tsp is on hand. How many teaspoons are required?

   a. .5 tsp
   b. 1 tsp
   c. 1.5 tsp
   d. 2 tsp

14. The physician ordered 10 units of regular insulin and 200 U/mL is on hand. How many milliliters are required?

   a. 0.05 mL
   b. 0.5 mL
   c. 1 mL
   d. 0.01 mL

15. The physician ordered 100 mg Ibuprofen/kg of body weight; on hand is 230 mg/tablet. The child weighs 50 lb. How many tablets are required?

   a. 1 tablet
   b. 5 tablets
   c. 10 tablets
   d. 15 tablets

16. The physician ordered 1,000 units of heparin; 5,000 U/mL is on hand. How many milliliters are required?

   a. 2 mL
   b. 0.2 mL
   c. 0.02 mL
   d. 1 mL

17. The physician ordered 5 mL of Kaopectate; 15 mL/tsp is on hand. How many teaspoons are required?

    a. 3 tsp
    b. 0.3 tsp
    c. 2 tsp
    d. 0.2 tsp

18. The physician orders 70 mg morphine sulphate; 1 g/mL is on hand. How many mL is required?

    a. 0.07 mL
    b. 0.7 mL
    c. 7 mL
    d. None of the Above

19. The physician ordered 200 mg amoxicillin to be given. The pharmacy stocks amoxicillin 400 mg per tsp. How many teaspoons are required?

    a. 1 tsp
    b. 0.5 tsp
    c. 1.5 tsp
    d. 2 tsp

20. The physician ordered 600 mg ibuprofen to be given now. The pharmacy stocks 200 mg per tablet. How many tablets are required?

    a. 1 tablet
    b. 2 tablets
    c. 3 tablets
    d. 4 tablets

Answer Key

1. A 0.5 mL
Dose ordered/Dose on hand X Quantity/1 = Required Dosage
40mg/80mg X 1 ML/1 = 40/80 =

2. B 0.5 tsp
Dose ordered/Dose on hand X Quantity/1 = Required Dosage
750 mg/1500mg X 1 tsp/1 = 750/1500 = 0.5 tsp

3. C 1.5 mL
Dose ordered/Dose on hand X Quantity/1 = Required Dosage
75mg/50mg X 1 mL/1 = 75/50 = 1.5 mL

4. B 1.5 tablets
Dose ordered/Dose on hand X Quantity/1 = Required Dosage
1500mg/1000mg X 1 tab/1 = 1500/1000 = 1.5 tablets

5. B 0.15 mL
Dose ordered/Dose on hand X Quantity/1 = Required Dosage
150 mg / 1000 mg X 1 mL/1 = 150/1000 = 0.15 mL
(Convert 1 g = 1000 mg)

6. D 0.1 mL
Dose ordered/Dose on hand X Quantity/1 = Required Dosage
10 units / 100 units X 1 mL / 1 = 10 / 100 = 0.1 mL

7. B 1 tablet
Dose ordered/Dose on hand X Quantity/1 = Required Dosage
5 mg / 5 mg X 1 tab / 1 = 5 / 5 = 1 tablet

8. A 3 tablets
Set up the formula to calculate the dose to be given in mg as per weight of the child:-

Dose ordered X Weight in Kg = Required Dose
20 mg X 12 kg = 240 mg

Dose ordered/Dose on hand X Quantity/1 = Required Dosage
240 mg / 80 mg X 1 tablet / 1 = 240 / 80 = 3 tablets

9. A 5 tablets
Set up the formula to calculate the dose to be given in mg as per weight of the child:

Dose ordered X Weight in Kg = Dose to be given

20 mg X 20 kg = 400 mg (Convert 44 lb to Kg, 1 lb = 0.4536 kg, hence 44 lb = 19.95 kg approx, 20 kg)

400 mg / 80 mg X 1 tablet / 1 = 400 / 80 = 5 tablets

10. D 0.6 mL
3000 units / 5000 units X 1 mL / 1 = 3000 / 5000 = 0.6 mL

11. B 0.75 mL
60 mg / 80 mg X 1 mL / 1 = 60 / 80 = 0.75 mL

12. C 3 tablets
Set up the formula to calculate the dose to be given in mg as per weight of the child:

Dose ordered X Weight in Kg = Required Dosage
16 mg X 15 kg = 240 mg

240 mg / 80 mg X 1 tablet / 1 = 240 = 3 tablets

13. B 1 tsp
Dose ordered X Weight in Kg = Required Dosage
Dose on hand: 1

1000 mg / 1000 mg X 1 tsp / 1 = 1000 / 1000 = 1 tsp
(Convert 1 g = 1000 mg)

14. A 0.05 mL

Dose ordered X Weight in Kg = Required Dosage
10 units / 200 units X 1 mL / 1 = 10 / 200 = 0.05 mL

15. C 10 tablets
Set up the formula to calculate the dose to be given in mg as per weight of the child:

Dose ordered X Weight in Kg = Required Dosage
100 mg X 23 kg = 2300 mg

(Convert 50 lb to Kg, 1 lb = 0.4536 kg, hence 50 lb = 50 X 0.4536 = 22.68 kg approx, 23 kg)

2300 mg / 230 mg X 1 tablet / 1 = 2300 / 230 = 10 tablets

16. B 0.2 mL
1000 units / 5000 units X 1 mL / 1 = 1000 / 5000 = 0.2 mL

17. A 3 tsp
5 mL / 15 mL X 1 tsp / 1 = 5 / 15 = 3 tsp

18. A 0.07 mL
70 mg / 1000 mg X 1 mL / 1 = 70 / 1000 = 0.07 mL
(Convert 1 g = 1000 mg)

19. B 0.5 tsp
200 mg / 400 mg X 1 tsp / 1 = 200 / 400 = 0.5 tsp

20. C 3 tablets
600 mg / 200 mg X 1 tablet / 1 = 600 / 200 = 3 tablets

Conclusion

CONGRATULATIONS! You have made it this far because you have applied yourself diligently to practicing for the exam and no doubt improved your potential score considerably! Getting into a good school is a huge step in a journey that might be challenging at times but will be many times more rewarding and fulfilling. That is why being prepared is so important.

Study then Practice and then Succeed!

Good Luck!

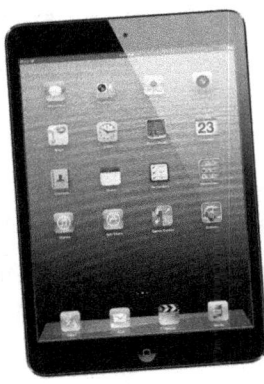

FREE Ebook Version

Download a FREE Ebook version of the publication!

Suitable for tablets, iPad, iPhone, or any smart phone.

Go to
http://tinyurl.com/lqn5w8y

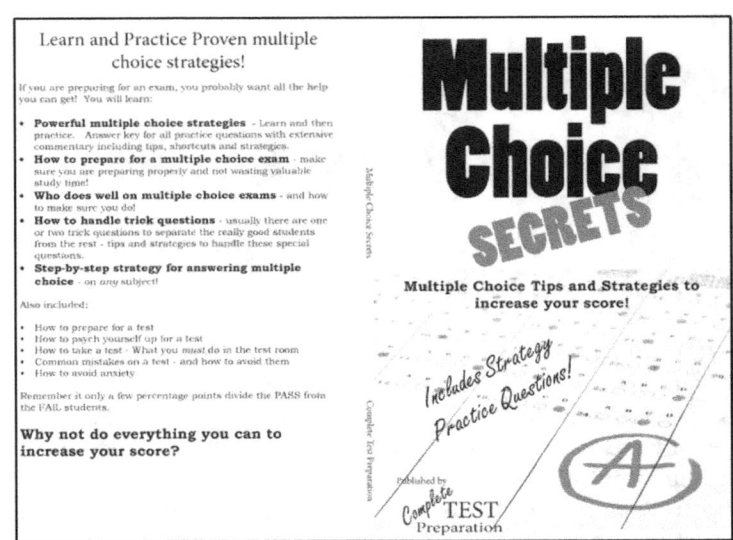

Multiple Choice Secrets!

Learn to increase your score using time-tested secrets for answering multiple choice questions!

This practice book has everything you need to know about answering multiple choice questions on a standardized test!

You will learn 12 strategies for answering multiple choice questions and then practice each strategy with over 45 reading comprehension multiple choice questions, with extensive commentary from exam experts!

Maybe you have read this kind of thing before, and maybe feel you don't need it, and you are not sure if you are going to buy this Book.

Even if our multiple choice strategies increase your score by a few percentage points, isn't that worth it?

Go to www.multiple-choice.ca start learning multiple choice secrets today!

Endnotes

[1] Mitosis. In *Wikipedia*. Retrieved November 12, 2010 from http://en.wikipedia.org/wiki/Mitosis

[2] Inegumentary. In *Wikipedia*. Retrieved November 12, 2010 from http://en.wikipedia.org/wiki/Integumentary

[3] Oncology. In *Wikipedia*. Retrieved November 12, 2010 from http://en.wikipedia.org/wiki/Oncology

[4] Medical Ethics In *Wikipedia*. Retrieved November 12, 2010 from http://en.wikipedia.org/wiki/Medical_ethics

[5] HCPCS. In *Wikipedia*. Retrieved November 12, 2010 from http://en.wikipedia.org/wiki/HCPCS

[6] Accounts Payable. In *Wikipedia*. Retrieved November 12, 2010 from http://en.wikipedia.org/wiki/Accounts_payable

[7] HCPCS Level 2 In *Wikipedia*. Retrieved November 12, 2010 from http://en.wikipedia.org/wiki/HCPCS_Level_2

[8] Controlled Substances Act. In *Wikipedia*. Retrieved November 12, 2010 from http://en.wikipedia.org/wiki/Controlled_Substances_Act

[9] http://en.wikipedia.org/wiki/File:SinusRhythmLabels.svg

[10] http://en.wikipedia.org/wiki/File:Axillary_lines.png

[11] Mandated Reporter. In *Wikipedia*. Retrieved November 12, 2010 from http://en.wikipedia.org/wiki/Mandated_reporter

[12] Managed Care. In *Wikipedia*. Retrieved November 12, 2010 from http://en.wikipedia.org/wiki/Managed_care

[13] Medication Errors. In *Wikipedia*. Retrieved November 12, 2010 from http://en.wikipedia.org/wiki/Medication_errors

[14] Medical Billing. In *Wikipedia*. Retrieved November 12, 2010 from http://en.wikipedia.org/wiki/Medical_billing_(United_States)

Images

[1] ECG Color. In *Wikipedia*. Retrieved November 12, 2010 from http://en.wikipedia.org/wiki/File:ECGcolor.svg

[2] ECG Color. In *Wikipedia*. Retrieved November 12, 2010 from http://en.wikipedia.org/wiki/File:ECGcolor.svg

www.ingramcontent.com/pod-product-compliance
Lightning Source LLC
Chambersburg PA
CBHW071826080526
44589CB00012B/927